Asbestos-related Diseases

Edited by Takemi Otsuki

Published in London, United Kingdom

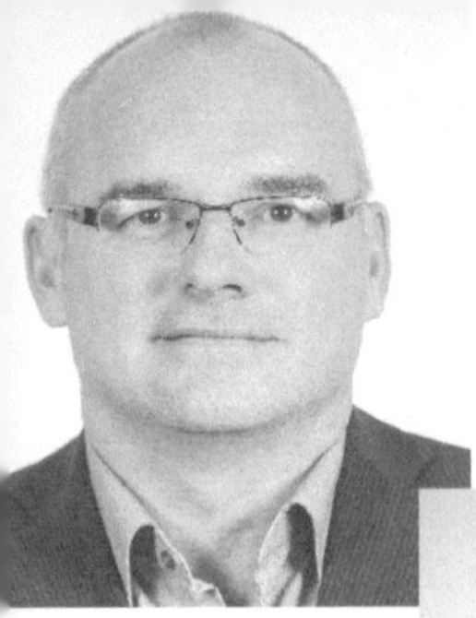
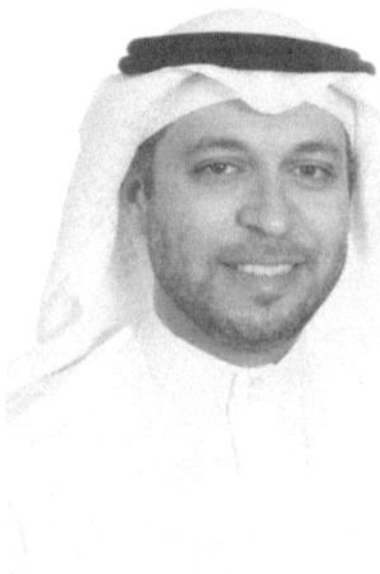
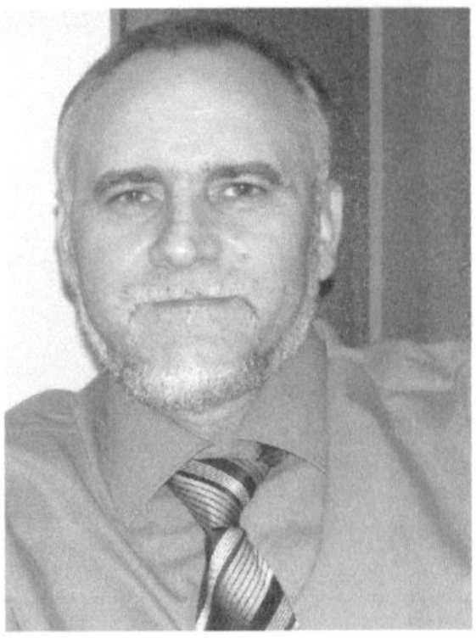
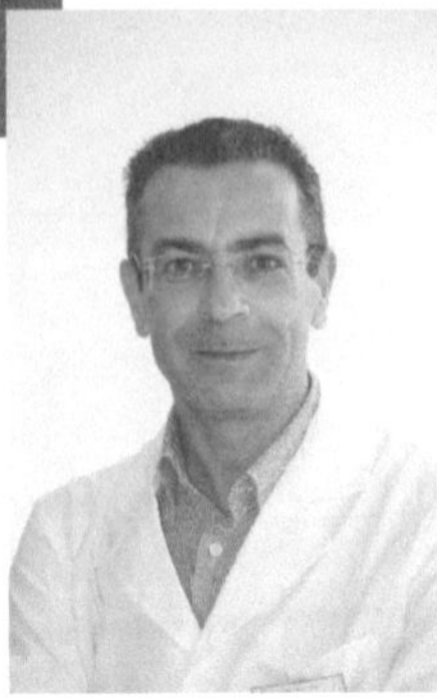
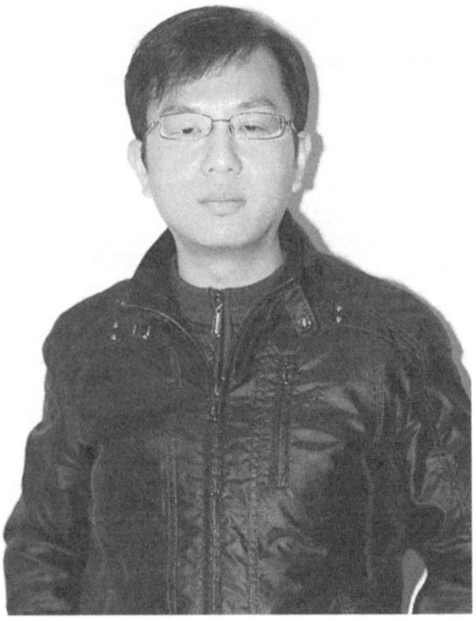
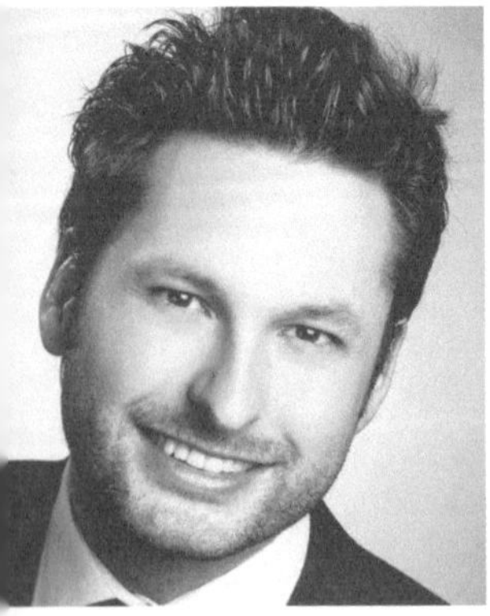
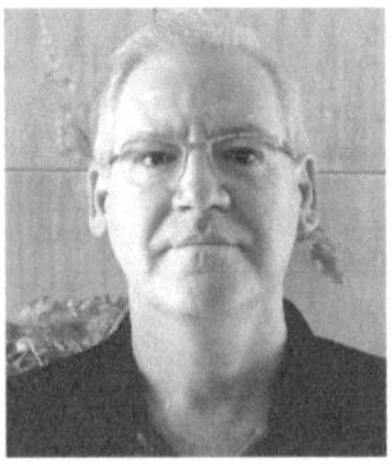

IntechOpen

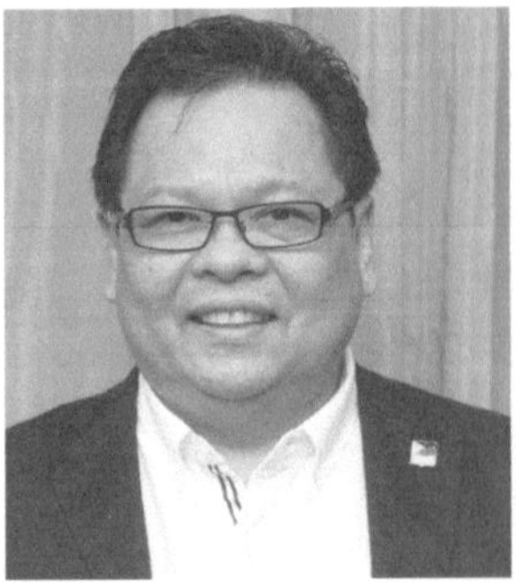
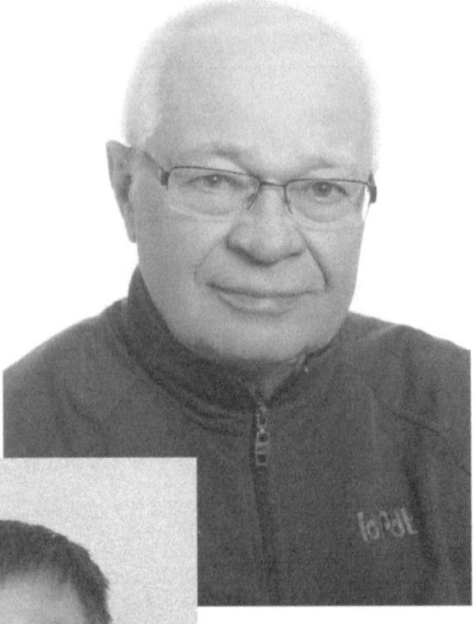
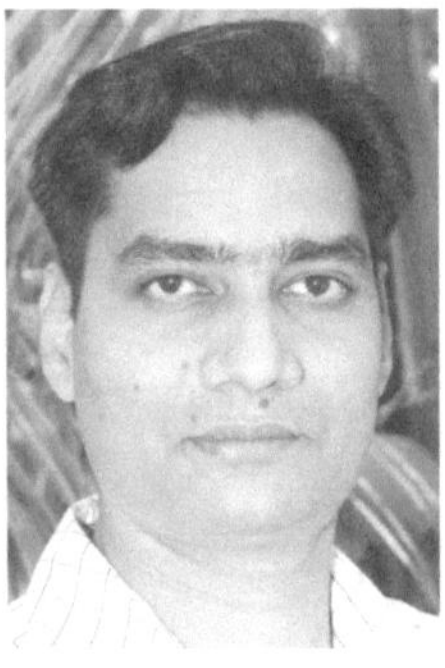
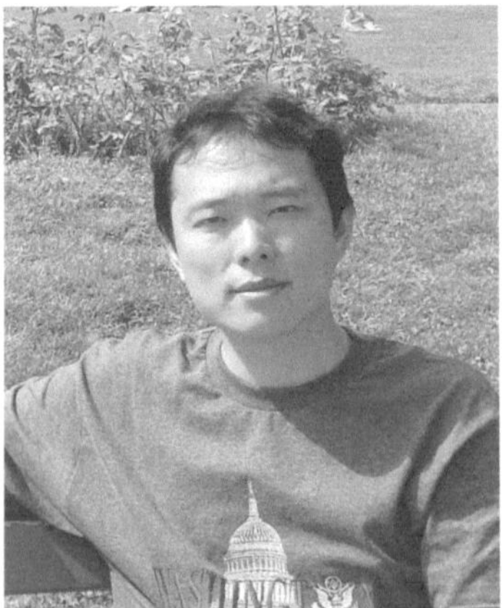
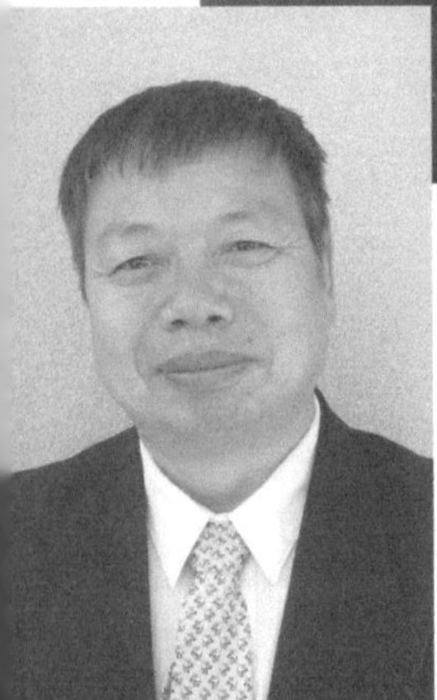
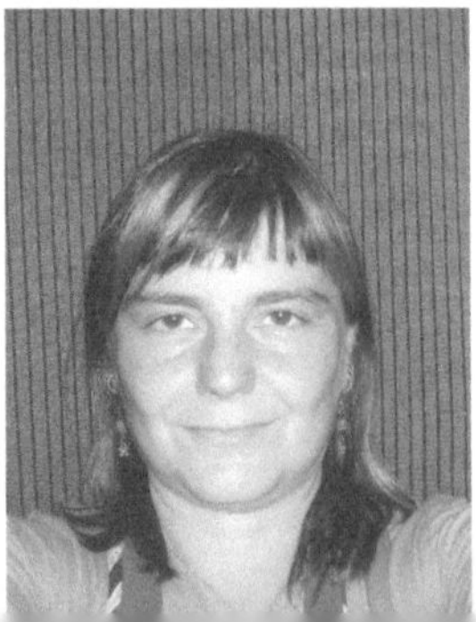

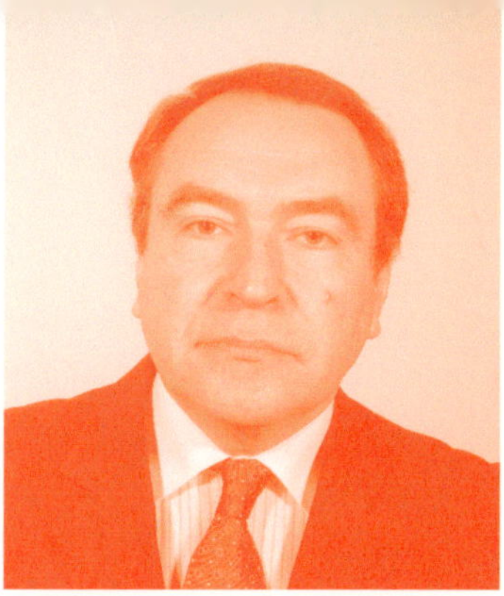
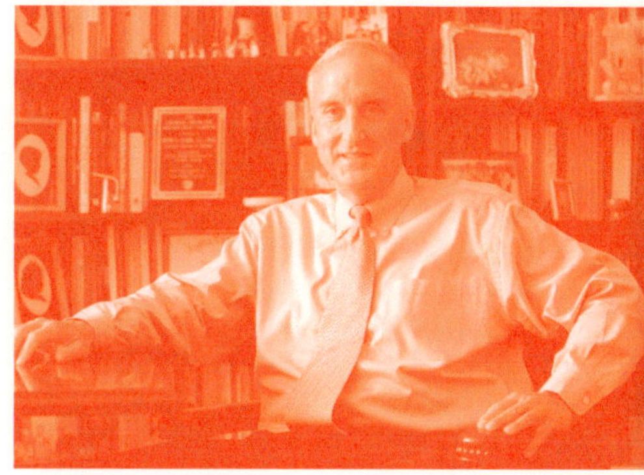
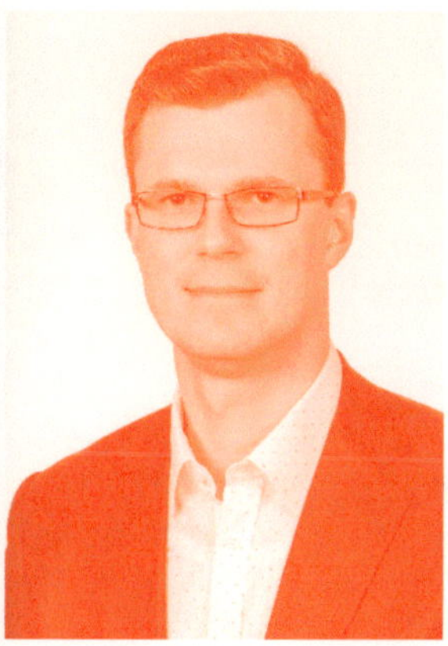
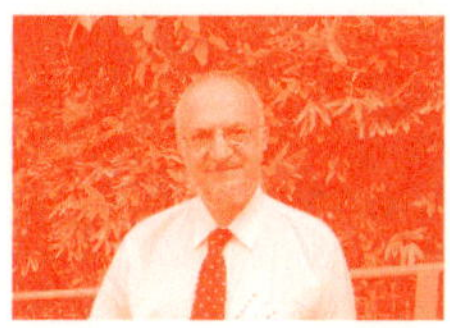
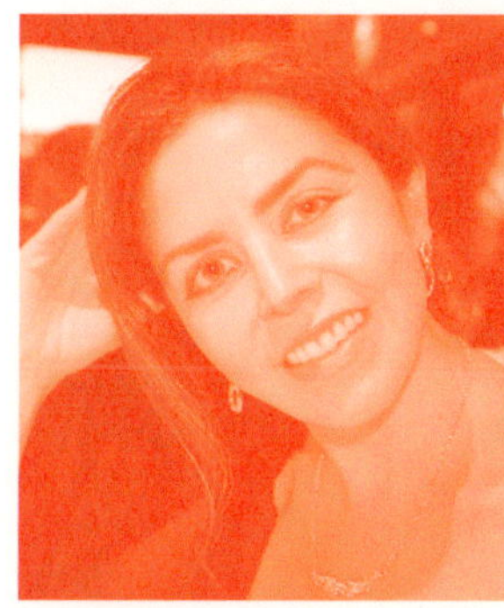

Supporting open minds since 2005

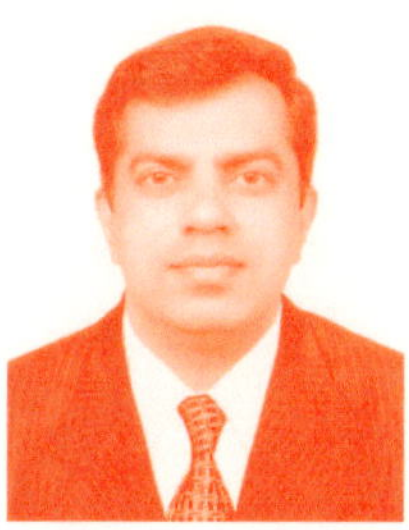
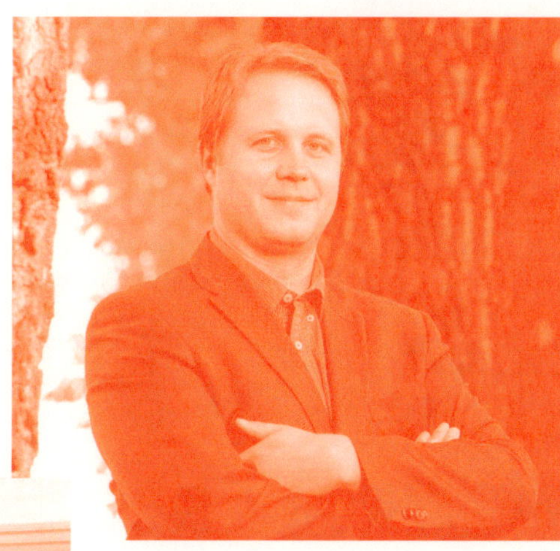
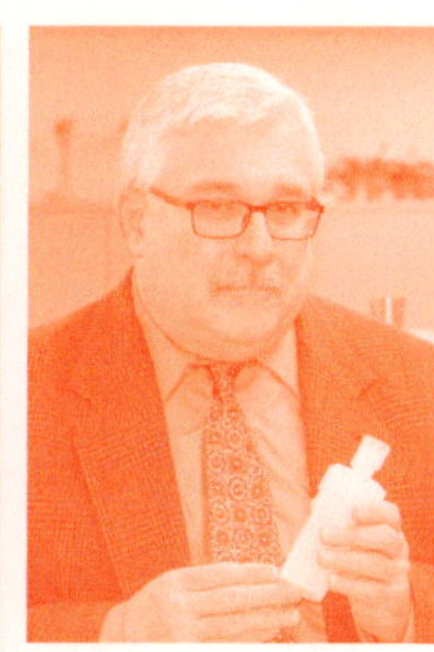
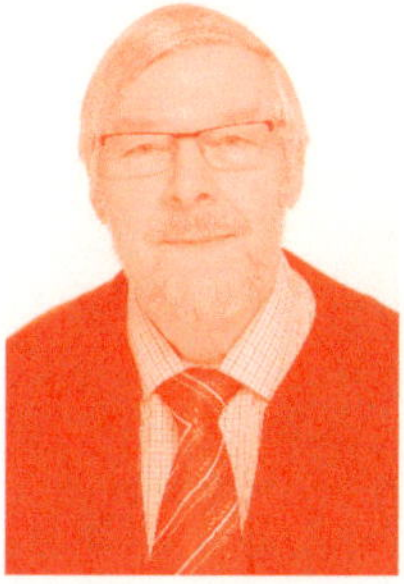
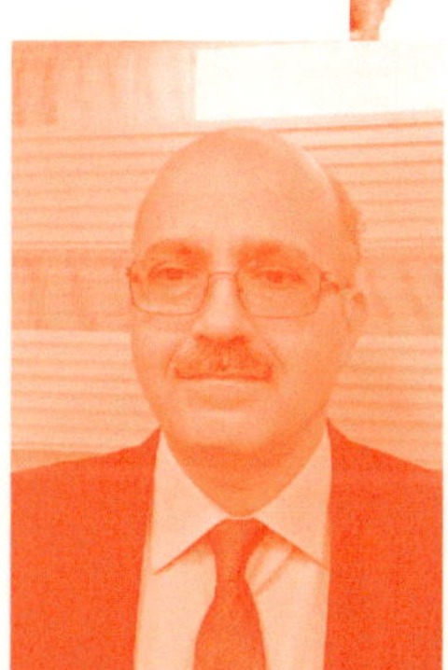
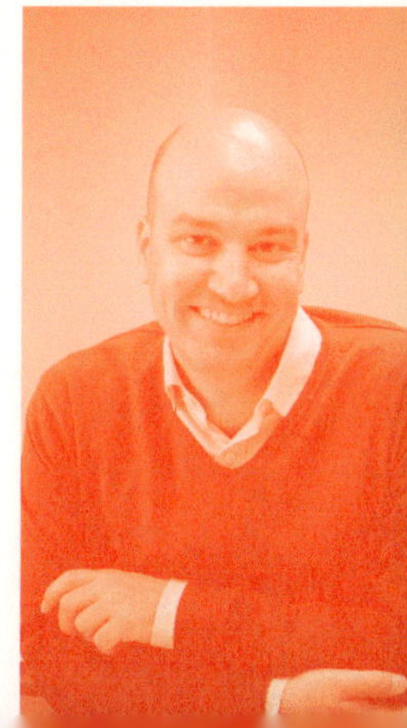
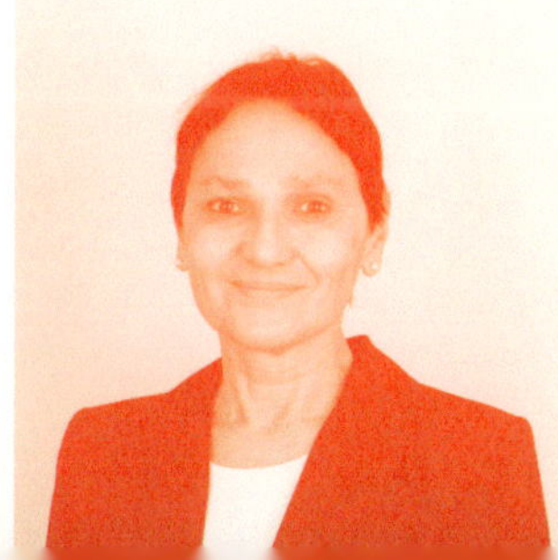

Asbestos-related Diseases
http://dx.doi.org/10.5772/intechopen.83098
Edited by Takemi Otsuki

Contributors
Shibo Ying, Yanbin Wang, Lyuyang Lyu, Yasumitsu Nishimura, Takemi Otsuki, Naoko Kumagai-Takei, Suni Lee, Kei Yoshitome, Yoshinori Kawabata, Nobukazu Fujimoto, Alenka Franko, Vita Dolžan, Katja Goricar, Metoda Dodic Fikfak

First published in London, United Kingdom, 2020 by IntechOpen
IntechOpen is the global imprint of INTECHOPEN LIMITED, registered in England and Wales, registration number: 11086078, 7th floor, 10 Lower Thames Street, London, EC3R 6AF, United Kingdom
Printed in Croatia

British Library Cataloguing-in-Publication Data
A catalogue record for this book is available from the British Library

Additional hard and PDF copies can be obtained from orders@intechopen.com

Asbestos-related Diseases
Edited by Takemi Otsuki
p. cm.
Print ISBN 978-1-83880-832-7
Online ISBN 978-1-83880-833-4
eBook (PDF) ISBN 978-1-83880-834-1

Meet the editor

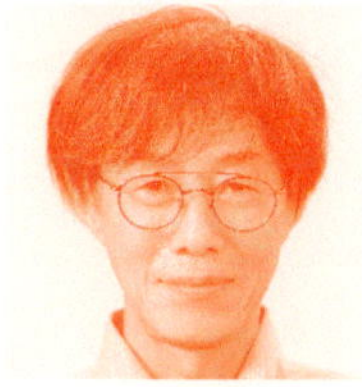

Prof. Takemi Otsuki graduated from Kawasaki Medical School (KMS), Kurashiki, Japan, in 1981. He then joined the Department of Hematology. In 1986, at the Institute of Medical Sciences, University of Tokyo, he was involved in clinical and experimental research in bone marrow transplantation. The theme of the post-graduate school (1985–1989) was myeloma cell biology. After joining the Department of Hematology, University of Minnesota (USA), in 1992, Dr. Otsuki studied genes involved in chromosomal translocations of lymphomas in the Department of Hematopathology at the US National Cancer Institute. He returned to the Department of Hygiene, KMS, in 1996 and became a professor there in 2003. Dr. Otsuki is engaged in research on health-promoting living environments as well as on the biological effects of fibrous particulate matter, especially on immune effects.

Contents

Preface

Asbestos-related issues are a major international concern, and the World Health Organization (WHO) has issued a declaration to eliminate asbestos-related diseases. However, there are still countries that export asbestos, and some countries have not banned its use. Considering that asbestos-related diseases, such as refractory and refractory malignant mesothelioma, will develop 30 to 50 years after the first exposure, the issue of asbestos-related diseases is of great importance.

Dr. Otsuki has been studying the immune effects of asbestos for 20 years. In observing the immunological effects of asbestos fibers, he, along with Associate Professor Nishimura, obtained research results that asbestos fibers bring about a reduction in antitumor immunity to various immunocompetent cells. This poses a challenge for the treatment of malignant mesothelioma using the immune checkpoint agent described in this text. Although there are biomarkers that can be used to detect asbestos exposure, there is currently only one way to detect pleural plaque and this is with radiological techniques. However, there are cases in which mesothelioma is discovered without sufficient discovery. In terms of cost, it is expensive to continuously screen members of high-risk groups of exposure (e.g., current or past workers in asbestos-handling factories, building demolition business, rubble disposal, etc.).

This book describes the immunological effects of asbestos fibers, biomarkers for malignant mesothelioma, pathology and clinical practice (especially the effects of immune checkpoints), and matrix metallopreteinases (MMPs).

This book is a useful reference for those who are involved in clinical and research studies of asbestos-induced diseases, as well as legislation and all other related areas.

Takemi Otsuki
Professor,
Department of Hygiene,
Kawasaki Medical School,
Kurashiki, Japan

Chapter 1

Suppressed Immune System Caused by Exposure to Asbestos and Malignant Mesothelioma

Yasumitsu Nishimura, Naoko Kumagai-Takei, Suni Lee, Kei Yoshitome and Takemi Otsuki

Abstract

Mesothelioma is the most serious of the asbestos-related diseases. It is caused by exposure to relatively low doses of asbestos and takes a long period to develop, which suggests the enactment of gradual adverse effects other than cellular toxicity. The immune system, which can play a role in tumor prevention, is a presumable target of asbestos by accumulation in lymph nodes and then slowly affecting functions of immune cells. Here, we describe key findings obtained from our studies concerning the immune-suppressive effects of asbestos and functional alteration in immune cells of patients with mesothelioma as well as plaque-positive subjects. Asbestos exposure of cell cultures resulted in decreased natural and acquired cytotoxicity exerted by NK cells and CTLs and the ability of Th1 cells to activate and support antitumor immunity. In contrast, asbestos exposure augmented Treg cell function and generation of fibrogenic/suppressive macrophages. Mesothelioma patients also showed similar characteristics in certain alterations caused by asbestos exposure. Additionally, our recent study established immunological screening devices for mesothelioma and asbestos exposure on the basis of comprehensive analysis of peripheral blood. Those findings underscore the importance of the immunological effects of asbestos and should assist further understanding of the mechanism and early detection of mesothelioma.

Keywords: macrophage, NK cell, Th1, Treg, CTL

1. Introduction: immune system as a key player in malignant mesothelioma following exposure to asbestos

Although asbestos has been banned in many European countries and the USA, as well as Japan, it continues to be used globally, and a report in 2018 by the WHO estimated that about 125 million people in the world continue to be exposed to asbestos at the workplace [1]. Occupational exposure to asbestos causes the death of at least 107,000 people from lung cancer, malignant mesothelioma, and pneumoconiosis (asbestosis) every year. Additionally, countries where asbestos remains have an increasing number of newly exposed individuals, especially during activities related to the destruction of old houses and buildings made of materials including some kinds of asbestos. That type of exposure to asbestos can occur in a variety of contexts such as the illegal destruction of asbestos-containing structures, the aftermath of natural disasters such as earthquakes and tsunamis, or even terrorism. It is known that the terrorist attacks in New York City on September 11, 2001, released 2000 tons of asbestos fibers into the air, subjecting an estimated 410,000 people to those fibers, including first responders, nearby residents, and workers in charge with cleaning up [2]. In the case of malignant mesothelioma, a poor prognostic disease specifically caused by the inhalation of asbestos, the disease develops silently and suddenly after about 40 years following the initial commencement of asbestos exposure, which means that deaths from malignant mesothelioma are increasing or achieving a peak in asbestos-banned countries. It has been estimated by Murayama T. that those deaths in Japan will peak around the year 2030 [3].

Thus, malignant mesothelioma is a global issue that needs to be solved. However, the following characteristics of mesothelioma make early diagnosis difficult to achieve. Malignant mesothelioma does not follow a dose-dependent rule in terms of toxicology but rather develops in people exposed to asbestos at low or middle doses of concentration [4]. Additionally, as mentioned above, it takes about 40 years to develop it. Therefore, sometimes people are suddenly informed that they have malignant mesothelioma, even though they do not remember any exposure to asbestos in their history, thereby leading to a delay in diagnosis. In the context of these characteristics of the relationship between asbestos exposure and malignant mesothelioma, we arrived at one possibility: alterations in immune functions might connect asbestos exposure to malignant mesothelioma. It is true that asbestos fibers cause cellular toxicity, mutagenicity, and the production of reactive oxygen species (ROS). Oxidized pyrimidine and alkalized nucleic acid base components correlate with the time of asbestos exposure, and the mutation frequency of lung DNA increased following intratracheal instillation of rats with asbestos [5–9]. Those findings indicate that asbestos fibers have the potential to cause transformation of healthy mesothelial cells. However, the body is equipped with an immune system, which can detect and remove those abnormal cells transiently arising due to certain kinds of toxic effects. Therefore, it is reasonable to assume that the immune system plays a role in protecting the body from malignant mesothelioma following exposure to asbestos and that the immune system must be subject to some kind of impairment prior to the development of mesothelioma. In fact, inhaled particles and fibers reach draining lymph nodes, and it has been reported that people exposed to asbestos occupationally or nonoccupationally showed accumulation of asbestos fibers in their lymph nodes [10, 11]. It is possible for asbestos to accumulate in the body slowly at low doses of exposure, thus subjecting immune cells to chronic asbestos exposure. Those cells circulate through the peripheral blood which might then result in a suppressed immune system. Moreover, if some alterations in the immune system are observed upon exposure to asbestos as well as in patients with malignant mesothelioma, we might utilize those changes to establish immunology-based screening devices to assist in the early detection of malignant mesothelioma as well as in cases of general asbestos exposure. Thus, we believe that the immune system is a key player in the mechanism involving asbestos-induced malignant mesothelioma and therefore a prime target for the development of screening methodologies. Consequently, we have been investigating the immunological effects of asbestos exposure and immunological alterations in patients with malignant mesothelioma and in people exposed to asbestos using multiple analyses of peripheral blood. Here we present the results of our investigations in this field and finally propose immunological screening devices for the detection of mesothelioma and asbestos exposure.

2. TGF-beta production by macrophages is crucial for suppressed antitumor immunity/tumor progression as well as lung fibrosis following asbestos exposure

Macrophages are the first population of immune cells which interact with inhaled asbestos in the body. It is well-known that alveolar macrophages (AMs) play a role in inflammation following inhalation of asbestos, where AM-mediated activities include the generation of reactive oxygen species (ROS), reactive nitrogen species (RNS), and inflammatory cytokines such as TNF-α [12–16]. Those inflammatory responses continue chronically since inhaled asbestos accumulates in the lungs, which induces overproduction of the extracellular matrix (ECM) and leads to asbestos-induced lung fibrosis, known as asbestosis [6, 17]. TNF-α chronically produced by AMs is a key phenomenon upstream of fibrosis because it induces production of transforming growth factor-beta (TGF-β) by fibroblasts and other cells, which in turn induces production of ECM. In fact, it has been reported that TNF-α-deficient mice showed decreased TGF-β as well as ECM following exposure to asbestos [17, 18]. Additionally, we also demonstrated in a previous study that the macrophage cell lines of RAW264.7 and J774 showed production of O_2^- and NO_2^- upon exposure to asbestos [14].

Thus, it is not unexpected that AMs have received attention given their role in inflammatory responses upon exposure to asbestos. However, we decided to focus on the fact that AMs also have the potential to produce TGF-β and that AMs can migrate away from the local site with chronic inflammation to other areas, where they are able to exert their effect in the absence of asbestos, which is more crucial for the induction of fibrogenic responses than simple production of TGF-β only at inflammatory sites. First, we noted that high doses of asbestos caused apoptosis of AMs during culture, while low doses failed to do so but did induce production of TGF-β. Therefore, we compared the ex vivo production of TGF-β by AMs from rats instilled with asbestos via the trachea with the in vitro production of TGF-β by AMs during culture upon exposure to asbestos. AMs collected at 5 days after instillation of rats with asbestos showed significantly higher amounts of TGF-β production in the culture for 5 days than AMs collected from control rats. However, it was surprising that AMs collected from control rats showed the same amount of TGF-β in the 5-day culture as AMs collected from rats exposed to asbestos in vivo. Moreover, AMs came to produce much greater amounts of TGF-β during continuous culture in fresh medium, and these viable AMs upon exposure to asbestos showed increased intracellular expression of Bcl-2, the product of a representative anti-apoptotic gene [19]. Those findings indicate that asbestos-exposed AMs can acquire the ability to produce high amounts of TGF-β in the absence of other cell types and with long survival supported by an anti-apoptotic gene, which might contribute to the progression of lung fibrosis following exposure to asbestos. That study was originally performed from the viewpoint of investigating the fibrogenic role of AMs as mentioned above. However, we believe that this functional alteration in AMs upon exposure to asbestos can be meaningfully interpreted as antitumor immunity upon exposure to asbestos. TGF-β is a representative cytokine that functions to suppress cell proliferation and survival of immune cells, natural killer (NK) cell function, and generation of cytotoxic T lymphocytes (CTLs) specific for tumors, as well as function in the induction of regulatory T cells [20–28]. TGF-β is produced by lymphoid cells as well as myeloid lineage cells, and those myeloid-derived suppressor cells play a role in angiogenesis which leads to tumor promotion [29]. Taken together, our findings underscore the significance of TGF-β production by macrophages which is crucial for suppressed antitumor immunity and tumor progression as well as lung fibrosis following asbestos exposure.

3. Impaired cytotoxicity of NK cells with altered expression of activating receptors caused by asbestos related with mesothelioma

NK cells represent one population of cells involved in innate immunity and play a role in tumor-surveillance as a first line of defense. One previous study has reported that people with low natural cytotoxic activity of peripheral blood lymphocytes showed higher cumulative incidence rates of cancer diseases than people with high activity in both men and women [30]. This highlights the importance of NK cell function in the prevention of tumor diseases including malignant mesothelioma following asbestos exposure. NK cells have a different machinery to recognize target cells compared with T lymphocytes. NK cells equip activating and inhibitory receptors against ligands expressed on the cell surface of targets, thereby determining whether or not to attack targets [31–37]. Finally, activating receptors engage in signal transduction to degranulate cytotoxic granules, including perforin and granzymes, which cause apoptosis of target cells [38]. Therefore, we focused on the effect of asbestos exposure on the expression of receptors on NK cells. First, we commenced continuous exposure of human NK cell line YT-A1 culture to asbestos. Following 1 month of culture, YT-A1 cells did not show any alterations in natural cytotoxic activity as measured by incubation with K562 cells. However, cells showed marked decreases in cytotoxicity after 4–5 months of culture with asbestos. It was also found that intracellular levels of granzyme A and perforin decreased in cells cultured with asbestos at the same time, but granzyme B did not decrease [39]. Furthermore, YT-A1 cells continuously exposed to asbestos (YT-CB5) showed decreases in cell surface expression of activating receptors NKG2D and 2B4 but did not show any alterations in the expression of NKG2A or CD94, which form a heterodimer that functions as an inhibitory receptor. NKG2D and NKG2A are members of the NKG2 family, members of which contain a lectin-like domain, whereas 2B4 (CD244) is a representative member of the signaling lymphocytic activation molecule (SLAM) family expressed on NK cells [32, 34]. Since NKG2D is known to contribute to natural cytotoxicity against K562 cells [40], it is reasonable to suggest that decreased cytotoxicity of YT-CB5 can be attributed to low expression of NKG2D. Signals from many activating receptors are mediated by extracellular signal-regulated kinase (ERK) and c-Jun N-terminal kinase (JNK) to effect degranulation [40]. In fact, it was found that YT-CB5 showed decreases in degranulation as well as phosphorylation of ERK1/2 following stimulation with antibodies to NKG2D [41]. 2B4 can receive stimulation with CD48 as ligand or anti-2B4 antibody to generate a signal that leads to cytotoxicity [35–37]. As 2B4 is not involved in the cytotoxicity of K562 cells, we utilized P815 cells bound to anti-2B4 antibody as targets to measure cytotoxicity with 2B4 receptor. It was found that YT-CB5 showed decreases in cytotoxicity against those P815 cells and in the degranulation induced by plate-coated antibodies to 2B4 [39]. Those findings indicate that asbestos exposure causes impaired cytotoxicity of NK cells attributable to alterations in cell surface expression of activating receptors. Moreover, we also examined the effect of asbestos exposure on NK cells using human peripheral blood mononuclear cells (PBMCs). Unlike the result obtained from cultures of YT-A1, NK cells in PBMC culture upon exposure to asbestos showed clear decreases in cell surface expression of NKp46 but not in NKG2D or 2B4 compared with grass wool representative man-made mineral fiber. NKp46 is a member of the natural cytotoxicity receptor (NCR) family, and it is known that the density of NKp46 is correlated with cytotoxicity against K562 cells [32–34]. Finally, we examined the natural cytotoxicity and expression of activating receptors of NK cells in PBMCs prepared from healthy volunteers and patients with malignant mesothelioma. Interestingly,

NK cells of mesothelioma patients showed low natural cytotoxicity as well as low expression of NKp46, but not of NKG2D or 2B4 in a similar manner to NK cells in PBMC culture exposed to asbestos. Taken together, our investigations of NK cell functions indicate that exposure to asbestos has the potential to decrease expression of activating receptors on NK cells, where NKp46 is a representative target for the effects of asbestos exposure, in addition to the NK cells of patients with malignant mesothelioma.

4. Decrease in Th1 phenotype caused by asbestos exposure and shown in mesothelioma patients more strongly than plaque-positive subjects

In an effort to examine the effect of asbestos exposure on $CD4^+$ T lymphocytes, our study utilized the human polyclonal T-cell line MT-2 [42, 43], and cells were cultured with continuous exposure to asbestos. From those cultures we obtained six asbestos-exposed sublines (MT-2CA1-3, MT-2CB1-3) and the original control MT-2 cell line (MT-2Org). Those cell lines were subjected to DNA microarray assays followed by clustering analyses. From the results, it was found that expression of 84 genes increased and 55 genes decreased by ca. twofold in the asbestos-exposed sublines and that all of the asbestos-exposed cell lines showed similar gene expression patterns [44]. Pathway and network analysis using the MetaCore System clarified that the Top 30 pathway results included the IFN-γ signaling pathway. Additionally, our previous study also identified decreases in IFN-γ production by MT-2CB1 cells [45]. In fact, the asbestos-exposed sublines showed decreases in expression of IFN regulatory factor 9 (IRF9) and IFN-stimulated gene factor-3 (ISGF3) as well as a chemokine receptor of CXCR3, which is positively regulated by IRF9. Th1 cells induced by stimulation are known to show increases in IFN-γ production and CXCR3 expression, which contribute to antitumor immune function [46, 47]. Flow cytometric analyses and real-time PCR (RT-PCR) confirmed that the percentage of cells positive for CXCR3 and mRNA levels of CXCR3 decreased in asbestos-exposed sublines, whereas that of CCR5, another chemokine receptor of the Th1-type, remained unchanged [44]. Moreover, $CD4^+$ T lymphocytes prepared from PBMCs were cultured in a similar manner upon exposure to asbestos. First, freshly purified $CD4^+$ T cells were expanded by stimulation with CD3 and CD28 to obtain sufficient cell numbers, and then those cells were utilized for culture in media supplemented with IL-2 upon exposure to asbestos. After 7 days of culture, there was no difference in $\%CXCR3^+$ cells between cultures with and without asbestos exposure, although the percentage of those cells decreased 28 days later, in contrast to no changes being observed in $\%CCR5^+$ cells. Additionally, asbestos-exposed $CD4^+$ T cells also showed decreases in intracellular expression of IFN-γ. Those findings are consistent with the results obtained from the experiment with MT-2 and indicate that asbestos exposure has the potential to effect a decrease in Th1 cell function of human primary T helper cells [48]. Finally, PBMCs from patients with malignant mesothelioma and subjects positive for pleural plaque, a representative sign of asbestos inhalation [5], were analyzed in a manner similar to the in vitro experiments mentioned above. Compared with healthy volunteers, both mesothelioma and plaque-positive groups showed low $\%CD4^+CXCR3^+$ cell numbers in PBMCs and were much lower in the mesothelioma than in the plaque-positive group, whereas $\%CD4^+CCR5^+$ numbers did not differ among the groups. Additionally, the mesothelioma group (but not the plaque-positive group) showed lower IFN-γ mRNA levels in $CD4^+$ T cells compared with healthy people [48]. Taken together, the results obtained from our studies demonstrate that asbestos exposure causes decreases in the Th1 phenotype of $CD4^+$ T cells, which is shown in patients with malignant mesothelioma more strongly than in plaque-positive subjects.

5. Augmented Treg function mediated through cell–cell interaction and suppressive cytokines caused by exposure to asbestos

Treg cells represent a key population of cells with the phenotype $CD4^+CD25^+Foxp3^+$ and function to suppress excess activation of immune responses as well as allow tumor cells to escape from immune surveillance [49, 50]. It has been reported that MT-2 cells also show this phenotype of cell surface markers and Treg-like suppressive function [51–54]. Additionally, MT-2 is a human polyclonal T-cell line immortalized by human T-cell leukemia virus type-1 (HTLV-1) and infection which causes adult T-cell leukemia (ATL) [42, 43]. Most $CD4^+CD25^+$ ATL cells express Foxp3, and some ATL cells have Treg-like suppressive function [51, 52, 54–56]. As a result, it has been suggested that ATL cells are derived from Treg cells. Therefore, MT-2 is useful in examining Treg cell function as well as Th cell function. Accordingly, we examined the Treg cell function of the MT-2 cell line continuously exposed to asbestos in the same manner as described above. First, we determined that the production of IL-10 increased twofold in the cell line exposed to asbestos relative to the original cell line, while the production of IFN-γ, TNF-α, and IL-6 decreased. IL-10 and TGF-β are immune-suppressive cytokines produced by Treg cells [26]. To examine phenomena upstream of the increase in IL-10 production, cells were treated with PP2, a specific inhibitor of Src family kinases (SFKs) which positively control IL-10 through transcription factors [57–59]. PP2 suppressed IL-10 mRNA levels, resulting in no difference between asbestos-exposed and nonexposed MT-2 sublines. Additionally, the subline exposed to asbestos showed increased Bcl-2 mRNA levels and a decrease in Bax, consistent with the fact that those cells survived in the toxic environment induced by exposure to asbestos. In fact, bcl-2 siRNA caused a decrease in cell growth upon exposure to asbestos. Moreover, phosphorylation of STAT3, part of the signaling pathway downstream of stimulation with IL-10 and target transcription of the bcl-2 gene, increased in the MT-2 subline exposed to asbestos [45]. Those findings indicate that asbestos induced an SFK-mediated increase in production of IL-10, in other words increased "Treg function," with increased survival ability attributed to high bcl-2 expression through the STAT pathway downstream of IL-10 in an autocrine manner. Furthermore, MT-2 subline exposed to asbestos was analyzed for Treg function in terms of suppressing the proliferation of $CD4^+CD25^-$ responder T (Tresp) cells, to express GITR and CTLA-4 cell surface markers and to produce suppressive cytokines such as TGF-β as well as IL-10. The asbestos-exposed subline showed enhanced suppression of Tresp cell proliferation stimulated with anti-CD3 antibody and induced dendritic cells (DCs), whereas there were no differences in cell proliferation stimulated with anti-CD3 and anti-CD28 antibodies between the sublines, suggesting the importance of cell–cell interactions for the enhanced suppression. Consistent with those findings, it was found that MT-2 subline exposed to asbestos tended to have decreased cell surface CTLA-4, which exerts suppressive function by cell–cell interactions with CD80 or CD86 on DCs [60, 61]. Additionally, TGF-β was produced at high concentrations by MT-2 subline exposed to asbestos, as IL-10 was also produced. It is interesting that the inhibited production of IL-10 or TGF-β by shRNA for those cytokine genes decreased the suppression efficiency of Tresp cell proliferation in the culture with transwell, indicating the absence of cell–cell interactions. Taken together, our results indicate that exposure to asbestos causes augmentation of Treg function mediated through cell–cell interactions as well as the production of suppressive cytokines.

6. Interfered induction and maintenance of cytotoxic T lymphocyte activity caused by asbestos and shown in mesothelioma, but not plaque-positive, subjects

$CD8^+$ cytotoxic T lymphocytes (CTLs) play a crucial role in antitumor immunity where they function to attack tumor cells together with NK cells [62]. Both NK cells and CTLs utilize perforin and granzymes to attack targets [63]. However, in contrast to NK cells, CTLs need to be induced from naïve $CD8^+$ T cells by stimulation with antigen for activation, which occurs upon interaction with DCs as well as $CD4^+$ T lymphocytes in lymph nodes [64–67], where inhaled asbestos fibers accumulate as mentioned above. Therefore, we sought to examine the effect of asbestos exposure on the induction phase of functional CTLs following stimulation with antigen. The mixed lymphocyte reaction (MLR) is an experimental and useful method to induce cell-mediated immunity by culturing two kinds of whole immune cells that differ allogenically from each other, such as $CD8^+$ T as well as $CD4^+$ T cells and DCs. Therefore, we employed MLR by culturing PBMCs as responder with allogenically different and irradiated PBMCs as stimulator upon exposure to asbestos in an effort to examine a variety of characteristics such as cell proliferation, cytotoxicity for allogenic target cells, and cytokine production by $CD8^+$ T cells. Asbestos exposure during culture for MLR caused suppressed cytotoxic activity of CTLs with decreased proliferation of $CD8^+$ T cells and production of IFN-γ and TNF-α, representative cytokines produced by activated CTLs [68]. Additionally, those CTLs harvested from culture with asbestos showed decreases in CD25 and CD45RO and an increase in CD45RA, which are activated and antigen-encountered markers and naïve markers on the cell surface, respectively [69]. Moreover, it is possible that prolonged exposure to asbestos might affect the functional activity of CTLs following antigen stimulation. EBT-8 is a cell line established from large granular lymphocyte leukemia of T-cell origin and shows surface expression of CD2, CD3, CD8, HLA-DR, and T-cell receptor alpha/beta, which are characteristic of cytotoxic T lymphocytes. Therefore, we examined alterations in the function of EBT-8 cells continuously exposed to asbestos for greater than 1 month. EBT-8 cells exposed to asbestos showed decreases in the percentage of cells positive for intracellular perforin, but not granzyme B. Additionally, those cells showed significantly decreased production of IFN-γ following stimulation with anti-CD3 antibody compared with control cells [70]. Those findings indicate that asbestos exposure interfered with the induction of functional CTLs following stimulation with antigen and that prolonged exposure to asbestos disrupts the functionality of CTLs, thereby leading to decreases in cytotoxic potential as well as production of IFN-γ. Along with those studies, we examined the functionality of $CD8^+$ T cells in peripheral blood of patients with malignant mesothelioma and pleural plaque-positive subjects. Mesothelioma patients showed decreases in the percentage of stimulation-induced intracellular $perforin^+$, but not $granzyme^+$, cells in $CD8^+$ T cells compared with healthy people, whereas plaque-positive subjects did not show any decrease [71]. Taken together, our results indicate that asbestos exposure interferes with induction and maintenance of functional CTLs, similar to peripheral $CD8^+$ T cells of mesothelioma patients.

7. Conclusion

Thus, our studies clarified a number of characteristics pertaining to asbestos-induced immunological impairment in acquired immunity as well as in innate immunity, some of which were also actually observed in patients with malignant mesothelioma. **Figure 1** summarizes those immune-suppressive effects of asbestos which presumably contribute to the development of malignant mesothelioma. Asbestos exposure suppressed immune-activating functions (Th1) and natural (NK) and acquired cytotoxicity (CTLs), whereas asbestos augmented functions of suppressive T lymphocytes (Tregs). Additionally, high production of TGF-β by long-surviving macrophages (Mϕ) caused by asbestos contributes to lung fibrosis as well as immune suppression. The immunological conditions generated by those characteristics allow abnormal cells caused by cellular toxicity of asbestos to escape from immune surveillance and survive to develop malignant mesothelioma. As mentioned above, it is actual that some of the characteristics caused by asbestos exposure were also shown in patients with malignant mesothelioma. Interestingly, plaque-positive subjects (without tumors) showed no impairment in some functions compared with mesothelioma patients, suggesting that their sustained immune functions protected them from malignant mesothelioma following asbestos exposure. On the basis of our present knowledge, we recently undertook a comprehensive analysis of the immunological characteristics of peripheral blood of mesothelioma patients as well as plaque-positive subjects. Parameters examined included cell surface markers, mRNA expression, and plasma cytokine concentrations. From the results of these analyses, we established three formulae for scoring mesothelioma, pleural plaque without tumors, and asbestos exposure (for both mesothelioma patients and plaque-positive subjects) (international patent

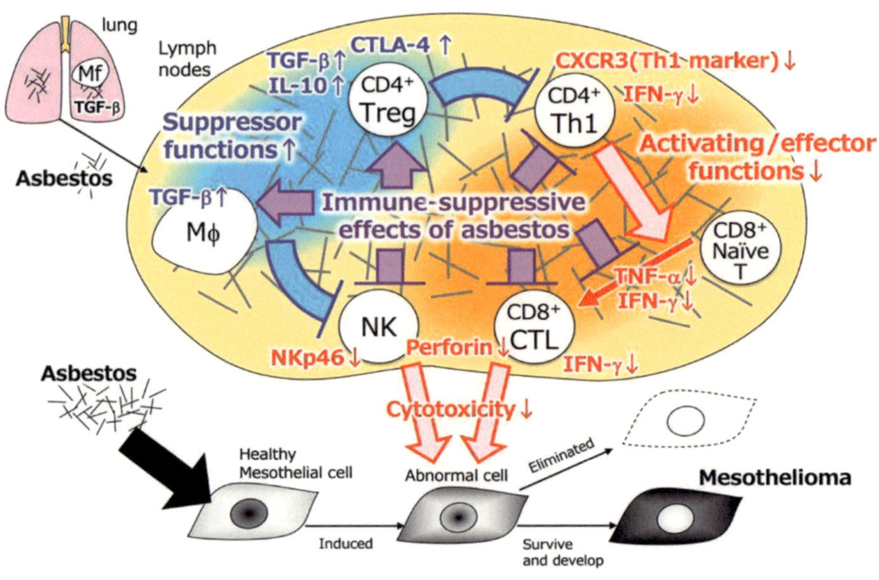

Figure 1.
Summarized illustration of the findings concerning a suppressed immune system caused by exposure to asbestos obtained from our studies. It was found that asbestos exposure showed immunological effects on various kinds of cells (purple arrows). Asbestos exposure during culture caused decreases in natural and acquired cytotoxicity and Th1 function associated with decreases in expression of NKp46, perforin, IFN-γ, TNF-α, and CXCR3 (colored red). In contrast, asbestos exposure caused increases in Treg function as well as fibrogenic/suppressive macrophages associated with increases in expression of CTLA-4, TGF-β, and IL-10 (colored blue). Those suppressed immune functions presumably allow abnormal mesothelial cells, arising from healthy cells caused by toxicity of asbestos, to escape from immune surveillance and survive to develop into malignant mesothelioma.

pending). The immunological screening devices might contribute to the detection of subgroups of people who have suppressed immune functions among people exposed to asbestos prior to diagnosis by CT images and histological observations. Moreover, those of our knowledge encourage us to treat mesothelioma with some kinds of immunotherapy. It is reasonable to assume that inhibitors targeting on Treg cells or suppressive macrophages might contribute to treatment of malignant mesothelioma. In addition, it has also been found that asbestos-caused decrease in cytotoxicity of CTL was improved by exogenous IL-2, but not accompanied with restoration of cell surface markers [72], which suggests that an appropriate immunotherapy might be developed to augment antitumor immunity in patients with mesothelioma as well as subjects exposed to asbestos. Thus, our studies could further our understanding of the immunological mechanisms associated with asbestos-induced malignant mesothelioma and perhaps facilitate the development of methodologies that can be employed for the early detection as well as treatment of mesothelioma. These are issues we intend to further address in the future.

Acknowledgements

The authors thank Ms. Tamayo Hatayama, Shoko Yamamoto, Miho Ikeda, and Ayasa Kamezaki for their technical assistance. Grant support from JPSS KAKENHI Grants (17790375, 18790386, 18390186, 19790411, 19790431, 20890270, 20390178, 22700933, 22790550, 23790679, 24590770, 25860470, 16 K09114, 16H05264, and 19H03892) and Kawasaki Medical School Project Grant (17-210S, 17-404 M, 18-209 T, 18-403, 19-205Y, 19-407 M, 20-210O, 20-411I, 21-107, 21-201, 21-401, 22-A29, 23B66, 23P3, and 28B051) is gratefully acknowledged.

Conflict of interest

The authors declare that there is no conflict of interest regarding the publication of this paper.

Author details

Yasumitsu Nishimura*, Naoko Kumagai-Takei, Suni Lee, Kei Yoshitome and Takemi Otsuki
Department of Hygiene, Kawasaki Medical School, Kurashiki, Japan

*Address all correspondence to: yas@med.kawasaki-m.ac.jp

References

[1] WHO. Asbestos: elimination of asbestos-related diseases; 2018. Available from: http://www.who.int/news-room/fact-sheets/detail/asbestos-elimination-of-asbestos-related-diseases

[2] King D. Asbestos, 9/11 and the World Trade Center; 2019. Available from: https://www.asbestos.com/world-trade-center/

[3] Murayama T, Takahashi K, Natori Y, Kurumatani N. Estimation of future mortality from pleural malignant mesothelioma in Japan based on an age-cohort model. American Journal of Industrial Medicine. 2006;**49**(1):1-7

[4] Bohlig H, Otto H. Asbest unt Mesotheliom : Fakten, Fragen, Umweltprobleme. Stuttgart: G. Thieme; 1975

[5] Sporn TA, Roggli VL. Mesothelioma. In: Roggli VL, Oury TD, Sporn TA, editors. Pathology of Asbestos-Associated Diseases. 3 Ed. New York: Springer-Verlag Berlin Heidelberg; 2014. pp. 81-140

[6] Mossman BT, Churg A. Mechanisms in the pathogenesis of asbestosis and silicosis. American Journal of Respiratory and Critical Care Medicine. 1998;**157**(5 Pt 1):1666-1680

[7] Mossman BT, Kamp DW, Weitzman SA. Mechanisms of carcinogenesis and clinical features of asbestos-associated cancers. Cancer Investigation. 1996;**14**(5):466-480

[8] Dusinska M, Collins A, Kazimirova A, Barancokova M, Harrington V, Volkovova K, et al. Genotoxic effects of asbestos in humans. Mutation Research. 2004;**553**(1-2):91-102

[9] Topinka J, Loli P, Georgiadis P, Dusinska M, Hurbankova M, Kovacikova Z, et al. Mutagenesis by asbestos in the lung of lambda-lacI transgenic rats. Mutation Research. 2004;**553**(1-2):67-78

[10] Dodson RF, Huang J, Bruce JR. Asbestos content in the lymph nodes of nonoccupationally exposed individuals. American Journal of Industrial Medicine. 2000;**37**(2):169-174

[11] Dodson RF, Williams MG Jr, Corn CJ, Brollo A, Bianchi C. A comparison of asbestos burden in lung parenchyma, lymph nodes, and plaques. Annals of the New York Academy of Sciences. 1991;**643**:53-60

[12] Kamp DW, Graceffa P, Pryor WA, Weitzman SA. The role of free radicals in asbestos-induced diseases. Free Radical Biology & Medicine. 1992;**12**(4):293-315

[13] Iguchi H, Kojo S, Ikeda M. Nitric oxide (NO) synthase activity in the lung and NO synthesis in alveolar macrophages of rats increased on exposure to asbestos. Journal of Applied Toxicology: JAT. 1996;**16**(4):309-315

[14] Nishiike T, Nishimura Y, Wada Y, Iguchi H. Production of nitric oxide elevates nitrosothiol formation resulting in decreased glutathione in macrophages exposed to asbestos or asbestos substitutes. Archives of Toxicology. 2005;**79**(2):83-89

[15] Dubois CM, Bissonnette E, Rola-Pleszczynski M. Asbestos fibers and silica particles stimulate rat alveolar macrophages to release tumor necrosis factor. Autoregulatory role of leukotriene B4. The American Review of Respiratory Disease. 1989;**139**(5):1257-1264

[16] Li XY, Lamb D, Donaldson K. The production of TNF-alpha and IL-1-like activity by bronchoalveolar leucocytes

after intratracheal instillation of crocidolite asbestos. International Journal of Experimental Pathology. 1993;**74**(4):403-410

[17] Liu JY, Brody AR. Increased TGF-beta1 in the lungs of asbestos-exposed rats and mice: Reduced expression in TNF-alpha receptor knockout mice. Journal of Environmental Pathology, Toxicology and Oncology: official organ of the International Society for Environmental Toxicology and Cancer. 2001;**20**(2):97-108

[18] Liu JY, Brass DM, Hoyle GW, Brody AR. TNF-alpha receptor knockout mice are protected from the fibroproliferative effects of inhaled asbestos fibers. The American Journal of Pathology. 1998;**153**(6):1839-1847

[19] Nishimura Y, Nishiike-Wada T, Wada Y, Miura Y, Otsuki T, Iguchi H. Long-lasting production of TGF-beta1 by alveolar macrophages exposed to low doses of asbestos without apoptosis. International Journal of Immunopathology and Pharmacology. 2007;**20**(4):661-671

[20] Ghiringhelli F, Menard C, Terme M, Flament C, Taieb J, Chaput N, et al. CD4+CD25+ regulatory T cells inhibit natural killer cell functions in a transforming growth factor-beta-dependent manner. The Journal of Experimental Medicine. 2005;**202**(8):1075-1085

[21] Gorelik L, Flavell RA. Immune-mediated eradication of tumors through the blockade of transforming growth factor-beta signaling in T cells. Nature Medicine. 2001;**7**(10):1118-1122

[22] Gorelik L, Flavell RA. Transforming growth factor-beta in T-cell biology. Nature Reviews. Immunology. 2002;**2**(1):46-53

[23] Li MO, Flavell RA. TGF-beta: A master of all T cell trades. Cell. 2008;**134**(3):392-404

[24] Li MO, Wan YY, Sanjabi S, Robertson AK, Flavell RA. Transforming growth factor-beta regulation of immune responses. Annual Review of Immunology. 2006;**24**:99-146

[25] Nakamura K, Kitani A, Strober W. Cell contact–dependent immunosuppression by Cd4+Cd25+regulatory T cells is mediated by cell surface–bound transforming growth factor β. The Journal of Experimental Medicine. 2001;**194**(5):629-644

[26] Shevach EM. Mechanisms of foxp3+ T regulatory cell-mediated suppression. Immunity. 2009;**30**(5):636-645

[27] Thomas DA, Massagué J. TGF-β directly targets cytotoxic T cell functions during tumor evasion of immune surveillance. Cancer Cell. 2005;**8**(5):369-380

[28] Trapani JA. The dual adverse effects of TGF-beta secretion on tumor progression. Cancer Cell. 2005;**8**(5):349-350

[29] Yang L, DeBusk LM, Fukuda K, Fingleton B, Green-Jarvis B, Shyr Y, et al. Expansion of myeloid immune suppressor gr+CD11b+ cells in tumor-bearing host directly promotes tumor angiogenesis. Cancer Cell. 2004;**6**(4):409-421

[30] Imai K, Matsuyama S, Miyake S, Suga K, Nakachi K. Natural cytotoxic activity of peripheral-blood lymphocytes and cancer incidence: An 11-year follow-up study of a general population. Lancet. 2000;**356**(9244):1795-1799

[31] Moretta A, Bottino C, Vitale M, Pende D, Cantoni C, Mingari MC, et al. Activating receptors and coreceptors involved in human natural killer cell-mediated cytolysis. Annual Review of Immunology. 2001;**19**:197-223

[32] Moretta L, Moretta A. Unravelling natural killer cell function: Triggering and inhibitory human NK receptors. The EMBO Journal. 2004;**23**(2):255-259

[33] Sivori S, Pende D, Bottino C, Marcenaro E, Pessino A, Biassoni R, et al. NKp46 is the major triggering receptor involved in the natural cytotoxicity of fresh or cultured human NK cells. Correlation between surface density of NKp46 and natural cytotoxicity against autologous, allogeneic or xenogeneic target cells. European Journal of Immunology. 1999;**29**(5):1656-1666

[34] Yokoyama WM, Plougastel BF. Immune functions encoded by the natural killer gene complex. Nature Reviews. Immunology. 2003;**3**(4):304-316

[35] Endt J, Eissmann P, Hoffmann SC, Meinke S, Giese T, Watzl C. Modulation of 2B4 (CD244) activity and regulated SAP expression in human NK cells. European Journal of Immunology. 2007;**37**(1):193-198

[36] Garni-Wagner BA, Purohit A, Mathew PA, Bennett M. Kumar V. A novel function-associated molecule related to non-MHC-restricted cytotoxicity mediated by activated natural killer cells and T cells. Journal of Immunology. 1993;**151**(1):60-70

[37] Valiante NM, Trinchieri G. Identification of a novel signal transduction surface molecule on human cytotoxic lymphocytes. The Journal of Experimental Medicine. 1993;**178**(4):1397-1406

[38] Trapani JA, Smyth MJ. Functional significance of the perforin/granzyme cell death pathway. Nature Reviews. Immunology. 2002;**2**(10):735-747

[39] Nishimura Y, Miura Y, Maeda M, Kumagai N, Murakami S, Hayashi H, et al. Impairment in cytotoxicity and expression of NK cell- activating receptors on human NK cells following exposure to asbestos fibers. International Journal of Immunopathology and Pharmacology. 2009;**22**(3):579-590

[40] Chen X, Trivedi PP, Ge B, Krzewski K, Strominger JL. Many NK cell receptors activate ERK2 and JNK1 to trigger microtubule organizing center and granule polarization and cytotoxicity. Proceedings of the National Academy of Sciences of the United States of America. 2007;**104**(15):6329-6334

[41] Nishimura Y, Maeda M, Kumagai N, Hayashi H, Miura Y, Otsuki T. Decrease in phosphorylation of ERK following decreased expression of NK cell-activating receptors in human NK cell line exposed to asbestos. International Journal of Immunopathology and Pharmacology. 2009;**22**(4):879-888

[42] Miyoshi I, Kubonishi I, Yoshimoto S. Shiraishi Y. A T-cell line derived from normal human cord leukocytes by co-culturing with human leukemic T-cells. Gann. 1981;**72**(6):978-981

[43] Miyoshi I, Kubonishi I, Yoshimoto S, Akagi T, Ohtsuki Y, Shiraishi Y, et al. Type C virus particles in a cord T-cell line derived by co-cultivating normal human cord leukocytes and human leukaemic T cells. Nature. 1981;**294**(5843):770-771

[44] Maeda M, Nishimura Y, Hayashi H, Kumagai N, Chen Y, Murakami S, et al. Reduction of CXC chemokine receptor 3 in an in vitro model of continuous exposure to asbestos in a human T-cell line, MT-2. American Journal of Respiratory Cell and Molecular Biology. 2011;**45**(3):470-479

[45] Miura Y, Nishimura Y, Katsuyama H, Maeda M, Hayashi H, Dong M, et al. Involvement of IL-10 and Bcl-2 in resistance against an

asbestos-induced apoptosis of T cells. Apoptosis: An International Journal on Programmed Cell Death. 2006;**11**(10):1825-1835

[46] Luster AD, Leder P. IP-10, a -C-X-C- chemokine, elicits a potent thymus-dependent antitumor response in vivo. The Journal of Experimental Medicine. 1993;**178**(3):1057-1065

[47] Sallusto F, Lanzavecchia A. Understanding dendritic cell and T-lymphocyte traffic through the analysis of chemokine receptor expression. Immunological Reviews. 2000;**177**:134-140

[48] Maeda M, Nishimura Y, Hayashi H, Kumagai N, Chen Y, Murakami S, et al. Decreased CXCR3 expression in CD4+ T cells exposed to Asbestos or derived from Asbestos-exposed patients. American Journal of Respiratory Cell and Molecular Biology. 2011;**45**(4):795-803

[49] Sakaguchi S. Naturally arising Foxp3-expressing CD25+CD4+ regulatory T cells in immunological tolerance to self and non-self. Nature Immunology. 2005;**6**(4):345-352

[50] Curotto de Lafaille MA, Lafaille JJ. Natural and adaptive foxp3+ regulatory T cells: More of the same or a division of labor? Immunity. 2009;**30**(5):626-635

[51] Shimauchi T, Kabashima K, Tokura Y. Adult T-cell leukemia/lymphoma cells from blood and skin tumors express cytotoxic T lymphocyte-associated antigen-4 and Foxp3 but lack suppressor activity toward autologous CD8+ T cells. Cancer Science. 2008;**99**(1):98-106

[52] Matsubar Y, Hori T, Morita R, Sakaguchi S, Uchiyama T. Delineation of immunoregulatory properties of adult T-cell leukemia cells. International Journal of Hematology. 2006;**84**(1):63-69

[53] Chen S, Ishii N, Ine S, Ikeda S, Fujimura T, Ndhlovu LC, et al. Regulatory T cell-like activity of Foxp3+ adult T cell leukemia cells. International Immunology. 2006;**18**(2):269-277

[54] Kohno T, Yamada Y, Akamatsu N, Kamihira S, Imaizumi Y, Tomonaga M, et al. Possible origin of adult T-cell leukemia/lymphoma cells from human T lymphotropic virus type-1-infected regulatory T cells. Cancer Science. 2005;**96**(8):527-533

[55] Karube K, Ohshima K, Tsuchiya T, Yamaguchi T, Kawano R, Suzumiya J, et al. Expression of FoxP3, a key molecule in CD4CD25 regulatory T cells, in adult T-cell leukaemia/lymphoma cells. British Journal of Haematology. 2004;**126**(1):81-84

[56] Roncador G, Garcia JF, Garcia JF, Maestre L, Lucas E, Menarguez J, et al. FOXP3, a selective marker for a subset of adult T-cell leukaemia/lymphoma. Leukemia. 2005;**19**(12):2247-2253

[57] Vega MI, Huerta-Yepaz S, Garban H, Jazirehi A, Emmanouilides C, Bonavida B. Rituximab inhibits p38 MAPK activity in 2F7 B NHL and decreases IL-10 transcription: Pivotal role of p38 MAPK in drug resistance. Oncogene. 2004;**23**(20):3530-3540

[58] Belkaid Y. Regulatory T cells and infection: A dangerous necessity. Nature Reviews. Immunology. 2007;**7**(11):875-888

[59] McGeachy MJ, Stephens LA, Anderton SM. Natural recovery and protection from autoimmune encephalomyelitis: Contribution of CD4+CD25+ regulatory cells within the central nervous system. Journal of Immunology. 2005;**175**(5):3025-3032

[60] Serra P, Amrani A, Yamanouchi J, Han B, Thiessen S, Utsugi T, et al. CD40 ligation releases immature dendritic cells from the control of regulatory

CD4+CD25+ T cells. Immunity. 2003;**19**(6):877-889

[61] Misra N, Bayry J, Lacroix-Desmazes S, Kazatchkine MD, Kaveri SV. Cutting edge: Human CD4+CD25+ T cells restrain the maturation and antigen-presenting function of dendritic cells. Journal of Immunology. 2004;**172**(8):4676-4680

[62] Banchereau J, Palucka AK. Dendritic cells as therapeutic vaccines against cancer. Nature Reviews. Immunology. 2005;**5**(4):296-306

[63] Harty JT, Tvinnereim AR, White DW. CD8+ T cell effector mechanisms in resistance to infection. Annual Review of Immunology. 2000;**18**:275-308

[64] Catalfamo M, Henkart PA. Perforin and the granule exocytosis cytotoxicity pathway. Current Opinion in Immunology. 2003;**15**(5):522-527

[65] Allan RS, Waithman J, Bedoui S, Jones CM, Villadangos JA, Zhan Y, et al. Migratory dendritic cells transfer antigen to a lymph node-resident dendritic cell population for efficient CTL priming. Immunity. 2006;**25**(1):153-162

[66] Weninger W, Manjunath N, von Andrian UH. Migration and differentiation of CD8+ T cells. Immunological Reviews. 2002;**186**:221-233

[67] Behrens G, Li M, Smith CM, Belz GT, Mintern J, Carbone FR, et al. Helper T cells, dendritic cells and CTL immunity. Immunology and Cell Biology. 2004;**82**(1):84-90

[68] Kumagai-Takei N, Nishimura Y, Maeda M, Hayashi H, Matsuzaki H, Lee S, et al. Effect of asbestos exposure on differentiation of cytotoxic T lymphocytes in mixed lymphocyte reaction of human peripheral blood mononuclear cells. American Journal of Respiratory Cell and Molecular Biology. 2013;**49**(1):28-36

[69] Fridman WH, Pages F, Sautes-Fridman C, Galon J. The immune contexture in human tumours: Impact on clinical outcome. Nature Reviews Cance. 2012;**12**(4):298-306

[70] Kumagai-Takei N, Nishimura Y, Matsuzaki H, Lee S, Yoshitome K, Otsuki T. Decrease in intracellular Perforin levels and IFN-γ production in human CD8+ T cell line following long-term exposure to Asbestos fibers. Journal of Immunology Research. 2018;**2018**:1-10

[71] Kumagai-Takei N, Nishimura Y, Maeda M, Hayashi H, Matsuzaki H, Lee S, et al. Functional properties of CD8(+) lymphocytes in patients with pleural plaque and malignant mesothelioma. Journal of Immunology Research. 2014;**2014**:670140

[72] Kumagai-Takei N, Nishimura Y, Matsuzaki H, Lee S, Yoshitome K, Hayashi H, et al. The suppressed induction of human mature cytotoxic T lymphocytes caused by Asbestos is not due to Interleukin-2 insufficiency. Journal of Immunology Research. 2016;**2016**:10

Chapter 2

Asbestos-Related Diseases and Blood Biomarkers

Alenka Franko, Vita Dolzan, Katja Goricar and Metoda Dodic Fikfak

Abstract

Asbestos-related diseases, including asbestosis, benign pleural diseases, lung cancer, other types of cancer, and especially malignant mesothelioma (MM), still represent an enormous problem all over the world and are among the most investigated occupational diseases. Considering that MM is a highly aggressive and severe malignant cancer of pleura, peritoneum and other serosal surfaces, new blood biomarkers for earlier diagnosis, following response to treatment and disease progression, have been intensively investigated. Several studies suggested that soluble mesothelin-related peptides, fibulin-3, survivin, osteopontin, vimentin, calretinin, and many others could be helpful in diagnosis, detecting the progression of MM and evaluating tumour response to treatment; however, these biomarkers have not been validated in clinical practice. Therefore, search for novel better stand-alone or composite biomarkers is under way. The aim of this chapter is to present the importance of blood biomarkers in evaluating the risk of developing asbestos-related diseases, early diagnosis, following the response to treatment and progression of these diseases, with special emphasis on MM.

Keywords: asbestos-related diseases, malignant mesothelioma, blood biomarkers

1. Introduction

Although the asbestos production and usage have been banned in many countries, the asbestos-related diseases still represent an enormous public health problem all over the world [1–3]. Occupational and environmental exposure to asbestos fibres has been associated with the development of asbestosis, pleural diseases such as pleural plaques, diffuse pleural thickening, pleural effusion, malignant mesothelioma (MM) of the pleura, peritoneum and other serosal surfaces, lung cancer, and some other types of malignant diseases, including cancer of the larynx, cancer of the ovary, and possibly also cancers of the buccal mucosa, the pharynx, the gastrointestinal tract, and the kidney [1–10]. The asbestos-related diseases are considered to be among the most investigated occupational diseases [1–3, 7, 8, 10]. In particular, MM, a highly aggressive cancer, causes serious concerns because of its dismal prognosis, poor therapeutic strategies, and fatality [11–13]. Therefore, search for novel better stand-alone or composite biomarkers is under way. This is especially important for high-risk populations with a known history of asbestos exposure.

The aim of this chapter is to present the importance of blood biomarkers in evaluating the risk of developing asbestos-related diseases, early diagnosis, following the response to treatment and progression of these diseases, with special emphasis on MM.

2. Blood biomarkers in asbestos-related diseases

It has been proposed that blood biomarkers, such as mesothelin, fibulin-3, osteopontin, vimentin, and many others, could enable noninvasive and early detection of asbestos-related diseases and could be particularly helpful in diagnosing MM, detecting the progression of this cancer and evaluating tumour response to treatment.

2.1 Mesothelin

One of the most investigated biomarkers in MM is mesothelin, a circulating form of a glycoprotein attached to the cell surface, that is considered to have a role in cell adhesion, proliferation, invasion, and possibly in cell-to-cell signalling. Mesothelin is highly expressed in MM as well as in several other cancers [14–18]. It exists in different forms that can be detected in serum in the form of soluble mesothelin-related peptides (SMRP) by enzyme-linked immunosorbent assay (ELISA) using monoclonal antibody techniques [19].Many studies have investigated mesothelin as a possible tumour biomarker for diagnosing MM, evaluating response to treatment, as well as for detecting the progression of this malignoma [16, 20–26].

Robinson et al. proposed SMRP as a marker for diagnosis and monitoring progression of the disease [20]. Later, the same group also suggested that SMRP may also be useful for monitoring MM progression and may prove useful for screening asbestos-exposed individuals for early MM [16].

Different mesothelin-related antibodies were tested in studies to detect different forms of mesothelin. Maeda et al. found that the soluble N-terminal fragment N-ERC/mesothelin is a very stable and plentiful in the blood [27]. Shiomi et al. identified N-ERC/mesothelin as a potential biomarker for MM and used newly developed ELISA system to gain data on N-ERC/mesothelin levels in different clinical settings. In their study, serum N-ERC/mesothelin levels showed that the median values from MM patients were extremely high as compared to levels obtained from other subjects (e.g., healthy volunteers and asbestos-related non-malignant diseases) [28].

Several other studies also reported higher levels of SMRP in subjects with MM and proposed that SMRP could be a useful tumour biomarker for diagnosing MM and monitoring the disease progression [21–24].

Franko et al. found that pre-treatment SMRP levels were significantly higher than in stable disease, partial response, and complete response, as were SMRP levels in progressive disease compared to stable disease, partial response, and complete response. The findings of this study also suggested that SMRP may be a useful tumour marker for detecting the progression of MM and evaluating tumour response to treatment [25].

A study of Hollevoet et al. investigated the diagnostic accuracy and use of serum mesothelin in early diagnosis by performing an individual patient data meta-analysis. The results of the study showed that in patients suspected of having MM, a positive blood test for mesothelin at a high-specificity threshold presented a strong incentive to urge further diagnostic steps. On the other hand, they reported that the poor sensitivity of mesothelin clearly limits its added value to early diagnosis [26].

The overall diagnostic accuracy of SMRPs in serum and the pleural fluid was also investigated in meta-analysis of Cui et al. [29]. The authors concluded that

SMRPs in serum and pleural fluid are helpful biomarkers for diagnosing MM, and that they have a similar diagnostic accuracy. However, they stressed that negative results of SMRP determinations are not sufficient to exclude MM, while the positive test results indicate that further invasive diagnostic steps might be necessary for the diagnosis of MM [29].

The meta-analysis by Gillezeau et al. studied the mean differences of mesothelin, osteopontin, and fibulin-3 in blood and pleural samples. A total of 32 studies with mesothelin levels were included. Statistically, significant mean differences have been found between MM patients and all the other comparison groups for mesothelin blood and pleural levels. It has been concluded that based on the findings, mesothelin levels seem to be significantly lower in all control groups compared with those with MM, suggesting a possible role of mesothelin as a screening biomarker for MM [30].

2.2 Fibulin

Human fibulin-3, also known as epidermal growth factor containing fibulin-like extracellular matrix protein 1 (EFEMP1), has also been investigated as a potential biomarker for asbestos-related diseases, especially for MM [31–33]. It is a member of a family of extracellular matrix glycoproteins [34] that have been proposed to be important in the regulation of cell proliferation and migration and to act as tumour suppressors or activators in different cancers [34–38]. Fibulin-3 is predominately localised in the extracellular matrix of elastic tissue, and it has restricted expression in the body [37].

Several studies showed that levels of fibulin-3 expression decreased in several types of cancer and were correlated with poor survival of patients with breast cancer [39], hepatocellular carcinoma [40], and lung cancer [41, 42]. On the contrary, an increase in fibulin-3 was found in cervical carcinomas [43], pancreatic cancer [44], and malignant gliomas [45].

Fibulin-3 was first investigated as a potential tumour biomarker of MM in the study of Pass et al. who found that plasma fibulin-3 levels can distinguish asbestos-exposed healthy persons from patients with MM [31]. Their results showed that plasma fibulin-3 levels in conjunction with fibulin-3 levels in pleural effusions can differentiate MM effusion from other malignant and benign effusions [31].

Several further studies investigated the possible role of fibulin-3 in the diagnosis of MM, but the results were not consistent. Kaya et al. proposed that real use of serum fibulin-3 was not for prognosis but for diagnosis of MM [46].

Ren et al. performed a systematic review and a meta-analysis of eight studies to evaluate the diagnostic value of fibulin-3 in plasma, serum, and pleural effusion. They found that the overall sensitivity and specificity for blood fibulin-3 were 0.87 [95% confidence interval (CI) 0.58-0.97] and 0.89 (95% CI 0.77-0.95), respectively. Based on these results, they concluded that fibulin-3 is a useful diagnostic biomarker for MM [47]. Similarly, Pei et al. reported that fibulin-3 confers a relatively high diagnostic efficacy and could be acceptable as an auxiliary biomarker to aid in MM identification [32].

Jiang et al. investigated the utility of fibulin-3 not only for MM but also for other asbestos-related diseases, therefore including patients with pleural plaques, asbestosis, and MM. The results showed that median plasma fibulin-3 level of subjects in the MM group was higher than that in other groups. The results also showed that subjects in the asbestosis group had a higher median fibulin-3 level compared to those in the control group. Their study proposed that fibulin-3 could be a potential biomarker for early screening of MM, but not for other asbestos-related diseases [33].

The meta-analysis of Gillezeau et al., which includes nine studies with fibulin-3 levels, also presented a statistically significant difference in both blood and pleural levels of fibulin-3 in MM patients compared with those of all other groups [30].

On the other hand, some other studies suggested that plasma fibulin-3 levels have low diagnostic accuracy [48–50]. The study of Creaney et al. identified soluble mesothelin as a superior diagnostic biomarker for MM compared to fibulin-3, whereas fibulin-3 provided superior prognostic information compared to mesothelin [48]. Kirschner et al. reported that plasma fibulin-3 level was significantly elevated in MM patients from the Sydney cohort, but not the Vienna cohort; however, the diagnostic accuracy was low. The data confirmed the potential prognostic value of pleural effusion fibulin-3 [49]. The same applies to the study of Ledda et al. who reported that fibulin-3 did not show a superior diagnostic performance [51].

The study of Kovac et al. aimed to evaluate the potential applicability of fibulin-3 plasma levels as a biomarker of response to treatment and its prognostic value for progressive disease within 18 months. The results of the study showed significantly higher fibulin-3 levels in progressive disease in comparison with the levels before treatment, in complete response to treatment, and in stable disease, which indicated that fibulin-3 could be helpful in identifying the progression of MM. On the contrary, no significant difference was observed between the fibulin-3 levels before treatment in comparison with the levels in complete response to treatment, partial response to treatment, and stable disease. The findings of this study suggest that fibulin-3 could be helpful in detecting the progression of MM [52].

2.3 Survivin

Survivin is a member of the inhibitor of the apoptosis protein (IAP) family and is known to have a role in the regulation of cell division and apoptosis (programmed cellular death). Survivin was first described as an inhibitor of caspase -9. However, several studies found that the role of survivin in pathogenesis of malignant diseases involves not only apoptosis but also the regulation of the mitotic spindle checkpoint, as well as chemoresistance and promotion of angiogenesis. This protein is commonly not expressed in normal differentiated tissues; however, it was found to be expressed in some cancers. Survivin is related to increased tumour aggressiveness, both in pleural fluid and in tissue [53].

Few studies investigated the role of survivin in asbestos-related diseases, or more precisely in MM. In their study, Hmeljak et al. performed on tissue samples aimed to elucidate whether survivin expression is associated with tumour cell proliferation and apoptosis and to investigate the prognostic and predictive value of survivin expression in MM. The results indicated that survivin expression might contribute to prediction of treatment response. However, the survivin expression in pleural MM did not show to have prognostic significance [54].

The only study so far that included blood (serum) samples is the study of Goricar et al. who investigated the influence of serum survivin levels on the outcome of cisplatin-based chemotherapy in patients with MM. The findings suggested that serum survivin levels could serve as a biomarker predicting response to treatment in MM before and during chemotherapy [55].

2.4 Osteopontin

Osteopontin is an extracellular cell adhesion protein that is involved in several biological processes, including cell-matrix interaction, cell-signalling and migration, immunological regulation, as well as in tumour development [56–60].

Elevated levels of serum osteopontin have been found in several cancers, such as colon cancer [61], breast cancer [62], lung cancer [63], as well as in MM [64]. Accordingly, serum osteopontin has been suggested to be a possible biomarker of early detection of MM [64–66].

Pass et al. investigated the presence of osteopontin in pleural MM and determined serum osteopontin levels in three populations: in asbestos-exposed subjects without cancer, subjects without cancer who were not exposed to asbestos, and in asbestos-exposed subjects with MM. Based on the results, the authors concluded that serum osteopontin levels could be used to distinguish asbestos-exposed individuals who do not have cancer from asbestos-exposed individuals with pleural MM [65].

The diagnostic performance of osteopontin was investigated in several other studies of asbestos-related diseases, but the results were not consistent [67–71].

Paleari et al. investigated the role of plasma osteopontin in diagnosis of pleural MM; however, their results suggested that plasma osteopontin levels cannot discriminate between chronic inflammatory and malignant lung disease [67].

The potential role of serum and plasma osteopontin in pleural MM diagnosis was reported by Cristaudo et al. [68]. Their results suggested that plasma osteopontin and serum osteopontin are not influenced by confounders such as age, smoking, and asbestos exposure. Moreover, plasma and serum osteopontin were proposed to be useful biomarkers in the diagnosis of epithelial MM in addition to radiological examination [68].

Comparison of plasma versus serum levels of osteopontin in patients with MM was performed by Creaney et al., who found that plasma osteopontin has a superior diagnostic accuracy to serum [69].

Osteopontin as the diagnostic biomarker was investigated in the cross-sectional study. The analysis showed that serum osteopontin levels in MM were higher than in benign asbestos-related diseases and healthy exposed subjects [70].

A systematic review and meta-analysis by Hu et al. aimed to evaluate the diagnostic accuracy of circulating osteopontin in pleural MM. Based on the analysis of six studies, the overall diagnostic sensitivity was 0.65 (95% CI 0.60–0.70) and specificity 0.81 (95% CI 0.78–0.85). The authors concluded that osteopontin is an effective marker for diagnosis of pleural MM [71].

Regarding peritoneal MM, osteopontin was studied as a potential circulating biomarker of diffuse peritoneal MM by Bruno et al. who reported that at multivariate analysis, osteopontin was related with survival. However, the authors concluded that osteopontin warrants further investigation as a prognostic marker for diffuse peritoneal MM [72].

Considering pleural plaques, Mastrangelo et al. investigated in their study whether plasma osteopontin was an indicator of asbestos exposure or effect. Their results suggested that osteopontin cannot be a reliable biomarker of asbestos exposure or effect (presence of pleural plaques) [73].

2.5 Calretinin

MM diagnosis is usually made at the advanced stages of the disease, which contributes to poor prognosis and short survival of MM patients [74, 75]. To confirm MM diagnosis, an immunohistochemical analysis investigating a panel of markers on tissue samples is required [75]. Among the positive immunohistochemical MM markers that can discriminate between malignant and mesothelial cells with the highest sensitivity and specificity are calretinin, cytokeratin5/6, and WT1 [76]. As biomarkers that would enable an earlier noninvasive diagnosis of MM are widely studied, recent studies evaluated if soluble calretinin could also be used as a biomarker in MM [75, 77–80].

Calretinin is a 30-kDa calcium-binding protein that belongs to the EF-hand family [81]. It acts as a calcium-buffering protein and calcium sensor. It plays an important role in the neurons, but it is also expressed in the mesothelial cells [81]. Calretinin was already shown to promote the invasiveness, proliferation, and migration of mesothelial cells [82]. It may also be involved in activating the focal adhesion kinase (FAK) signalling pathway and epithelial-to-mesenchymal transition [82].

Studies showed that calretinin was increased in plasma and serum of MM patients compared to patients with other asbestos-related diseases and healthy controls [75, 79, 80]. Interestingly, patients with asbestosis also had slightly higher serum calretinin compared to patients with pleural plaques [75]. The ELISA assay developed by Raiko et al. is highly sensitive when used to detect calretinin in plasma or serum and is robust enough to detect calretinin in retrospective samples regardless of storage time [75, 79]. However, as calretinin is mostly expressed in epithelioid and biphasic MM, but only in around 30% of sarcomatoid MM [81], its usefulness as a soluble biomarker is limited in this histological subtype [75].

Studies also suggest that using a combination of calretinin and mesothelin can increase the sensitivity for detecting MM [75, 77]. In asbestos-exposed subjects that developed MM, calretinin was increased already in prediagnostic plasma samples (even more than a year prior to the clinical diagnosis) compared to asbestos-exposed subjects that did not develop MM, especially in samples closer to the diagnosis [77]. Even though sensitivity was limited to an individual biomarker, using a combination of both calretinin and mesothelin had better predictive ability and could also be important as a screening biomarker in asbestos-exposed subjects [77].

2.6 Other biomarkers

Apart from the most frequently studied biomarkers described above, some studies investigated other serum or plasma factors in asbestos-related diseases [83–85]. Among protein biomarkers, megakaryocyte potentiating factor and high mobility group box 1 (HMGB1) were increased in MM patients compared to healthy individuals or patients with benign asbestos-related diseases [84, 85].

Additionally, novel studies suggest microRNA (miRNA) expression could also serve as a diagnostic or prognostic biomarker in MM [84–86]. Kirschner et al. compared cell-free miRNA profiles in plasma from MM patients with healthy controls and proposed the potential role of miRNA-29c* and miRNA-92a as a candidate tumour biomarkers, and indicated that miRNA-625-3p is a promising novel diagnostic marker for MM [86]. Micolucci et al. in their systematic review and a quantitative meta-analysis compared the data from asbestos-exposed and MM subjects and suggested that the most promising candidates for a multimarker signature were circulating miRNA-126-3p, miRNA-103a-3p, and miRNA-625-3p in combination with mesothelin [87]. Mozzoni et al. aimed to identify a pattern of miRNA (mi-RNA-16, miRNA-17, mi-RNA-126, and miRNA-486) as a possible diagnostic biomarker for patients with pleural MM and asbestosis and as prognostic biomarkers for patients with pleural MM. The results showed that all miRNA levels were decreased in patients with pleural MM or asbestosis, which has been suggested to support the role of circulating miRNAs as potential biomarkers for asbestos-related diseases. Additionally, miRNA-16 was directly related to prognosis of patients with pleural MM, indicating its possible use as prognostic factor in patients with pleural MM [88]. Santarelli et al. performed a study to identify miRNAs associated with asbestos-induced malignances. In this study, four serum miRNAs (mi-RNA-126, miRNA-205, miRNA-222, and miRNA-520g) were implicated in asbestos-related malignant diseases and could be utilised for screening in asbestos-exposed populations [89].

As individual biomarkers that have been proposed in asbestos-related diseases have some limitations, it was suggested that a combination of different factors might be a better diagnostic or prognostic biomarker in asbestos-related diseases [83–85].

3. The role of composite blood biomarkers in asbestos-related diseases

Several studies investigated the potential role of composite blood biomarkers in asbestos-related diseases, and many of them included mesothelin together with various other biomarkers [72, 90].

Felten et al. assessed the influence of age and asbestos exposure on the blood levels of the proposed tumour markers, mesothelin, and osteopontin and determined the change of these markers over time. The results showed that age had a strong influence on biomarker levels. On the other hand, there was no association between asbestos exposure duration or benign asbestos-related diseases and biomarker levels. The researchers concluded that fixed cut-off values for deciding between intensive clinical work-up and continued surveillance appeared inadequate for evaluating markers [91].

In addition to evaluating the potential applicability of fibulin-3 plasma levels as a biomarker of response to treatment and progression of disease, the study of Kovac et al. also assessed the potential applicability of fibulin-3 in comparison with or in addition to SMRP. The results indicated that in addition to SMRP, fibulin-3 could also be useful in detecting MM progression [52].

Bonotti et al. evaluated the usefulness of SMRP, plasma osteopontin, and vimentin as markers of the clinical response to treatment in patients suffering from epithelioid MM. In their study, SMRP, osteopontin, and vimentin showed statistically significant differences between the disease categories: stable disease, partial response, and disease progression. Based on the results, it has been concluded that the time course of SMRP and vimentin was strongly associated with disease status, and so was the time course of osteopontin, although to a lesser extent. The researchers suggested that these markers appear to be particularly effective in cases of partial response and disease progression, even though their possible use in stable disease should be better elucidated [90].

In a recent study that evaluated soluble mesothelin, calretinin, and megakaryocyte potentiating factor, the use of composite of these biomarkers improved the performance for diagnosis of pleural MM compared to population controls [78]. The combination of calretinin and megakaryocyte potentiating factor had the highest sensitivity in men, while the combination of calretinin and mesothelin had the highest sensitivity in women [78].

In an Italian cohort, the diagnostic performance of fibulin-3 against SMRP was compared in patients with pleural effusion from MM. The results of the study showed that the levels of fibulin-3 were similar in pleural effusions from pleural MM and pleural effusion from other pathologies in contrast to SMRP levels, which were significantly higher in pleural effusion from pleural MM. A further analysis confirmed that SMRP showed a good performance, whereas fibulin was not able to discriminate pleural MM from other pathologies. The conclusion was that fibulin detection in pleural effusion, contrary to SMRP detection, is not useful as a biomarker for the diagnosis of pleural effusion from pleural MM [92].

Bruno et al. assessed the diagnostic and prognostic values of mesothelin, osteopontin, CEA, CA19-9, CA125, and CA15-3 in diffuse peritoneal MM and other peritoneal malignancies. The conclusion was that when assessing peritoneal surface malignancies of unknown origin, elevated mesothelin with low CA19-9 may increase the suspicion index for diffuse peritoneal MM. As for the role of osteopontin, further research is needed [72].

4. Conclusions

Considering that asbestos-related diseases, and in particular MM, still represent a huge health problem and economic burden, the investigation of potential biomarkers for evaluating the risk for developing asbestos-related diseases, earlier diagnosis of asbestos diseases, evaluating respond to treatment and progression of these diseases, is of great importance. Biomarkers for assessing risk of developing asbestos diseases are of considerable significance especially in high asbestos-exposed populations. As presented in the chapter, the results of the studies are not consistent, therefore further research is needed to clarify inconsistency and find reliable biomarkers that could be used in clinical practice and would enable better outcome of asbestos-related diseases and increase survival in MM.

Author details

Alenka Franko[1,2]*, Vita Dolzan[3], Katja Goricar[3] and Metoda Dodic Fikfak[1,2]

1 Clinical Institute of Occupational Medicine, University Medical Centre, Ljubljana, Slovenia

2 Faculty of Medicine, University of Ljubljana, Slovenia

3 Pharmacogenetics Laboratory, Faculty of Medicine, Institute of Biochemistry, University of Ljubljana, Slovenia

*Address all correspondence to: alenka.franko@siol.net

References

[1] Stayner L, Welch LS, Lemen R. The worldwide pandemic of asbestos-related diseases. Annual Review of Public Health. 2013;**34**:205-216

[2] Takahashi K, Landrigan PJ, Collegium R. The global health dimensions of asbestos and asbestos-related diseases. Annals of Global Health. 2016;**82**(1):209-213

[3] Visona SD, Villani S, Manzoni F, Chen Y, Ardissino G, Russo F, et al. Impact of asbestos on public health: A retrospective study on a series of subjects with occupational and non-occupational exposure to asbestos during the activity of Fibronit plant (Broni, Italy). Journal of Public Health Research. 2018;**7**(3):1519

[4] Hillerdal G, Henderson DW. Asbestos, asbestosis, pleural plaques and lung cancer. Scandinavian Journal of Work, Environment & Health. 1997;**23**(2):93-103

[5] Cugell DW, Kamp DW. Asbestos and the pleura: A review. Chest. 2004;**125**(3):1103-1117

[6] Antao VC, Larson TC, Horton DK. Libby vermiculite exposure and risk of developing asbestos-related lung and pleural diseases. Current Opinion in Pulmonary Medicine. 2012;**18**(2):161-167

[7] Vainio H. Epidemics of asbestos-related diseases--something old, something new. Scandinavian Journal of Work, Environment & Health. 2015;**41**(1):1-4

[8] Marsili D, Terracini B, Santana VS, Ramos-Bonilla JP, Pasetto R, Mazzeo A, et al. Prevention of asbestos-related disease in countries currently using asbestos. International Journal of Environmental Research and Public Health. 2016;**13**(5):1-19

[9] Solbes E, Harper RW. Biological responses to asbestos inhalation and pathogenesis of asbestos-related benign and malignant disease. Journal of Investigative Medicine. 2018;**66**(4):721-727

[10] Dolzan V, Dodic-Fikfak M, Franko A. Gene-environment interactions: The case of asbestosis. In: Korhan O, editor. Occupational Health. Rijeka: InTech; 2017. pp. 159-178

[11] Robinson BWS, Lake RA. Medical progress - advances in malignant mesothelioma. The New England Journal of Medicine. 2005;**353**(15):1591-1603

[12] Miller JM, Thompson JK, MacPherson MB, Beuschel SL, Westbom CM, Sayan M, et al. Curcumin: A double hit on malignant mesothelioma. Cancer Prevention Research (Philadelphia, Pa.). 2014;**7**(3):330-340

[13] Rossini M, Rizzo P, Bononi I, Clementz A, Ferrari R, Martini F, et al. New perspectives on diagnosis and therapy of malignant pleural mesothelioma. Frontiers in Oncology. 2018;**8**:91

[14] Chang K, Pastan I. Molecular cloning of mesothelin, a differentiation antigen present on mesothelium, mesotheliomas, and ovarian cancers. Proceedings of the National Academy of Sciences of the United States of America. 1996;**93**(1):136-140

[15] Scholler N, Fu N, Yang Y, Ye Z, Goodman GE, Hellstrom KE, et al. Soluble member(s) of the mesothelin/megakaryocyte potentiating factor family are detectable in sera from patients with ovarian carcinoma. Proceedings of the National Academy of Sciences of the United States of America. 1999;**96**(20):11531-11536

[16] Robinson BW, Creaney J, Lake R, Nowak A, Musk AW, de Klerk N, et al. Soluble mesothelin-related protein--a blood test for mesothelioma. Lung Cancer. 2005;**49**(Suppl 1):S109-S111

[17] Tian L, Zeng R, Wang X, Shen C, Lai Y, Wang M, et al. Prognostic significance of soluble mesothelin in malignant pleural mesothelioma: A meta-analysis. Oncotarget. 2017;**8**(28):46425-46435

[18] He X, Wang L, Riedel H, Wang K, Yang Y, Dinu CZ, et al. Mesothelin promotes epithelial-to-mesenchymal transition and tumorigenicity of human lung cancer and mesothelioma cells. Molecular Cancer. 2017;**16**(1):63

[19] Peake MD, Entwisle J, Gray S. Malignant pleural mesothelioma: clinical presentation, radiological evaluation and diagnosis. In: O'Byrne K, Rusch V, editors. Malignant Pleural Mesothelioma. Oxford, New York: Oxford University Press; 2006. pp. 35-60

[20] Robinson BW, Creaney J, Lake R, Nowak A, Musk AW, de Klerk N, et al. Mesothelin-family proteins and diagnosis of mesothelioma. Lancet. 2003;**362**(9396):1612-1616

[21] Beyer HL, Geschwindt RD, Glover CL, Tran L, Hellstrom I, Hellstrom KE, et al. MESOMARK: A potential test for malignant pleural mesothelioma. Clinical Chemistry. 2007;**53**(4):666-672

[22] Scherpereel A, Grigoriu B, Conti M, Gey T, Gregoire M, Copin MC, et al. Soluble mesothelin-related peptides in the diagnosis of malignant pleural mesothelioma. American Journal of Respiratory and Critical Care Medicine. 2006;**173**(10):1155-1160

[23] Grigoriu BD, Scherpereel A, Devos P, Chahine B, Letourneux M, Lebailly P, et al. Utility of osteopontin and serum mesothelin in malignant pleural mesothelioma diagnosis and prognosis assessment. Clinical Cancer Research. 2007;**13**(10):2928-2935

[24] Cristaudo A, Foddis R, Vivaldi A, Guglielmi G, Dipalma N, Filiberti R, et al. Clinical significance of serum mesothelin in patients with mesothelioma and lung cancer. Clinical Cancer Research. 2007;**13**(17):5076-5081

[25] Franko A, Dolzan V, Kovac V, Arneric N, Dodic-Fikfak M. Soluble mesothelin-related peptides levels in patients with malignant mesothelioma. Disease Markers. 2012;**32**(2):123-131

[26] Hollevoet K, Reitsma JB, Creaney J, Grigoriu BD, Robinson BW, Scherpereel A, et al. Serum mesothelin for diagnosing malignant pleural mesothelioma: An individual patient data meta-analysis. Journal of Clinical Oncology. 2012;**30**(13):1541-1549

[27] Maeda M, Hino O. Molecular tumor markers for asbestos-related mesothelioma: Serum diagnostic markers. Pathology International. 2006;**56**(11):649-654

[28] Shiomi K, Hagiwara Y, Sonoue K, Segawa T, Miyashita K, Maeda M, et al. Sensitive and specific new enzyme-linked immunosorbent assay for N-ERC/mesothelin increases its potential as a useful serum tumor marker for mesothelioma. Clinical Cancer Research. 2008;**14**(5):1431-1437

[29] Cui A, Jin XG, Zhai K, Tong ZH, Shi HZ. Diagnostic values of soluble mesothelin-related peptides for malignant pleural mesothelioma: Updated meta-analysis. BMJ Open. 2014;**4**(2):e004145

[30] Gillezeau C, van Gerwen M, Ramos J, Liu B, Flores R, Taioli E. Biomarkers for malignant pleural mesothelioma: A meta-analysis. Carcinogenesis. 2019. DOI: 10.1093/carcin/bgz103. [Epub ahead of print]

[31] Pass HI, Levin SM, Harbut MR, Melamed J, Chiriboga L, Donington J, et al. Fibulin-3 as a blood and effusion biomarker for pleural mesothelioma. The New England Journal of Medicine. 2012;**367**(15):1417-1427

[32] Pei D, Li Y, Liu X, Yan S, Guo X, Xu X, et al. Diagnostic and prognostic utilities of humoral fibulin-3 in malignant pleural mesothelioma: Evidence from a meta-analysis. Oncotarget. 2017;**8**(8):13030-13038

[33] Jiang Z, Ying S, Shen W, He X, Chen J, Xia H, et al. Plasma fibulin-3 as a potential biomarker for patients with asbestos-related diseases in the han population. Disease Markers. 2017;**2017**:1725354

[34] Timpl R, Sasaki T, Kostka G, Chu ML. Fibulins: A versatile family of extracellular matrix proteins. Nature Reviews. Molecular Cell Biology. 2003;**4**(6):479-489

[35] Argraves WS, Greene LM, Cooley MA, Gallagher WM. Fibulins: Physiological and disease perspectives. EMBO Reports. 2003;**4**(12):1127-1131

[36] Kim IG, Kim SY, Choi SI, Lee JH, Kim KC, Cho EW. Fibulin-3-mediated inhibition of epithelial-to-mesenchymal transition and self-renewal of ALDH+ lung cancer stem cells through IGF1R signaling. Oncogene. 2014;**33**(30):3908-3917

[37] Kobayashi N, Kostka G, Garbe JH, Keene DR, Bachinger HP, Hanisch FG, et al. A comparative analysis of the fibulin protein family. Biochemical characterization, binding interactions, and tissue localization. The Journal of Biological Chemistry. 2007;**282**(16):11805-11816

[38] Zhang Y, Marmorstein LY. Focus on molecules: Fibulin-3 (EFEMP1). Experimental Eye Research. 2010;**90**(3):374-375

[39] Sadr-Nabavi A, Ramser J, Volkmann J, Naehrig J, Wiesmann F, Betz B, et al. Decreased expression of angiogenesis antagonist EFEMP1 in sporadic breast cancer is caused by aberrant promoter methylation and points to an impact of EFEMP1 as molecular biomarker. International Journal of Cancer. 2009;**124**(7):1727-1735

[40] Nomoto S, Kanda M, Okamura Y, Nishikawa Y, Qiyong L, Fujii T, et al. Epidermal growth factor-containing fibulin-like extracellular matrix protein 1, EFEMP1, a novel tumor-suppressor gene detected in hepatocellular carcinoma using double combination array analysis. Annals of Surgical Oncology. 2010;**17**(3):923-932

[41] Yue W, Dacic S, Sun Q, Landreneau R, Guo M, Zhou W, et al. Frequent inactivation of RAMP2, EFEMP1 and Dutt1 in lung cancer by promoter hypermethylation. Clinical Cancer Research. 2007;**13**(15 Pt 1): 4336-4344

[42] Xu S, Yang Y, Sun YB, Wang HY, Sun CB, Zhang X. Role of fibulin-3 in lung cancer: in vivo and in vitro analyses. Oncology Reports. 2014;**31**(1):79-86

[43] En-lin S, Sheng-guo C, Hua-qiao W. The expression of EFEMP1 in cervical carcinoma and its relationship with prognosis. Gynecologic Oncology. 2010;**117**(3):417-422

[44] Seeliger H, Camaj P, Ischenko I, Kleespies A, De Toni EN, Thieme SE, et al. EFEMP1 expression promotes in vivo tumor growth in human pancreatic adenocarcinoma. Molecular Cancer Research: MCR. 2009;**7**(2):189-198

[45] Hu B, Thirtamara-Rajamani KK, Sim H, Viapiano MS. Fibulin-3 is uniquely upregulated in malignant gliomas and promotes tumor cell

motility and invasion. Molecular Cancer Research: MCR. 2009;7(11):1756-1770

[46] Kaya H, Demir M, Taylan M, Sezgi C, Tanrikulu AC, Yilmaz S, et al. Fibulin-3 as a diagnostic biomarker in patients with malignant mesothelioma. Asian Pacific Journal of Cancer Prevention : APJCP. 2015;**16**(4):1403-1407

[47] Ren R, Yin P, Zhang Y, Zhou J, Zhou Y, Xu R, et al. Diagnostic value of fibulin-3 for malignant pleural mesothelioma: A systematic review and meta-analysis. Oncotarget. 2016;7(51):84851-84859

[48] Creaney J, Dick IM, Meniawy TM, Leong SL, Leon JS, Demelker Y, et al. Comparison of fibulin-3 and mesothelin as markers in malignant mesothelioma. Thorax. 2014;**69**(10):895-902

[49] Kirschner MB, Pulford E, Hoda MA, Rozsas A, Griggs K, Cheng YY, et al. Fibulin-3 levels in malignant pleural mesothelioma are associated with prognosis but not diagnosis. British Journal of Cancer. 2015;**113**(6):963-969

[50] Sun HH, Vaynblat A, Pass HI. Diagnosis and prognosis-review of biomarkers for mesothelioma. Annals of Translational Medicine. 2017;**5**(11):244

[51] Ledda C, Caltabiano R, Vella F, Matera S, Marconi A, Loreto C, et al. Fibulin-3 as biomarker of malignant mesothelioma. Biomarkers in Medicine. 2019;**13**(10):875-886

[52] Kovac V, Dodic-Fikfak M, Arneric N, Dolzan V, Franko A. Fibulin-3 as a biomarker of response to treatment in malignant mesothelioma. Radiology and Oncology. 2015;**49**(3):279-285

[53] Mita AC, Mita MM, Nawrocki ST, Giles FJ. Survivin: Key regulator of mitosis and apoptosis and novel target for cancer therapeutics. Clinical Cancer Research. 2008;**14**(16):5000-5005

[54] Hmeljak J, Erculj N, Dolzan V, Pizem J, Kern I, Kovac V, et al. Is survivin expression prognostic or predictive in malignant pleural mesothelioma? Virchows Archiv. 2013;**462**(3):315-321

[55] Goricar K, Kovac V, Franko A, Dodic-Fikfak M, Dolzan V. Serum survivin levels and outcome of chemotherapy in patients with malignant mesothelioma. Disease Markers. 2015;**2015**:316739

[56] Wai PY, Kuo PC. The role of Osteopontin in tumor metastasis. Journal of Surgical Research. 2004;**121**(2):228-241

[57] Frey AB, Wali A, Pass H, Lonardo F. Osteopontin is linked to p65 and MMP-9 expression in pulmonary adenocarcinoma but not in malignant pleural mesothelioma. Histopathology. 2007;**50**(6):720-726

[58] Ohashi R, Tajima K, Takahashi F, Cui R, Gu T, Shimizu K, et al. Osteopontin modulates malignant pleural mesothelioma cell functions in vitro. Anticancer Research. 2009;**29**(6):2205-2214

[59] Tajima K, Ohashi R, Sekido Y, Hida T, Nara T, Hashimoto M, et al. Osteopontin-mediated enhanced hyaluronan binding induces multidrug resistance in mesothelioma cells. Oncogene. 2010;**29**(13):1941-1951

[60] Chen RX, Xia YH, Xue TC, Ye SL. Osteopontin promotes hepatocellular carcinoma invasion by up-regulating MMP-2 and uPA expression. Molecular Biology Reports. 2011;**38**(6):3671-3677

[61] Coppola D, Szabo M, Boulware D, Muraca P, Alsarraj M, Chambers AF, et al. Correlation of osteopontin protein expression and pathological stage across a wide variety of tumor histologies. Clinical Cancer Research. 2004;**10**(1 Pt 1):184-190

[62] El-Tanani MK, Yuen HF, Shi Z, Platt-Higgins A, Buckley NE, Mullan PB, et al. Osteopontin can act as an effector for a germline mutation of BRCA1 in malignant transformation of breast cancer-related cells. Cancer Science. 2010;**101**(6):1354-1360

[63] Rouanne M, Adam J, Goubar A, Robin A, Ohana C, Louvet E, et al. Osteopontin and thrombospondin-1 play opposite roles in promoting tumor aggressiveness of primary resected non-small cell lung cancer. BMC Cancer. 2016;**16**:483

[64] Chen Z, Gaudino G, Pass HI, Carbone M, Yang H. Diagnostic and prognostic biomarkers for malignant mesothelioma: An update. Translational Lung Cancer Research. 2017;**6**(3):259-269

[65] Pass HI, Lott D, Lonardo F, Harbut M, Liu Z, Tang N, et al. Asbestos exposure, pleural mesothelioma, and serum osteopontin levels. The New England Journal of Medicine. 2005;**353**(15):1564-1573

[66] Ivanov SV, Ivanova AV, Goparaju CM, Chen Y, Beck A, Pass HI. Tumorigenic properties of alternative osteopontin isoforms in mesothelioma. Biochemical and Biophysical Research Communications. 2009;**382**(3):514-518

[67] Paleari L, Rotolo N, Imperatori A, Puzone R, Sessa F, Franzi F, et al. Osteopontin is not a specific marker in malignant pleural mesothelioma. The International Journal of Biological Markers. 2009;**24**(2):112-117

[68] Cristaudo A, Foddis R, Bonotti A, Simonini S, Vivaldi A, Guglielmi G, et al. Comparison between plasma and serum osteopontin levels: Usefulness in diagnosis of epithelial malignant pleural mesothelioma. The International Journal of Biological Markers. 2010;**25**(3):164-170

[69] Creaney J, Yeoman D, Musk AW, de Klerk N, Skates SJ, Robinson BW. Plasma versus serum levels of osteopontin and mesothelin in patients with malignant mesothelioma--which is best? Lung Cancer. 2011;**74**(1):55-60

[70] Bayram M, Dongel I, Akbas A, Benli I, Akkoyunlu ME, Bakan ND. Serum biomarkers in patients with mesothelioma and pleural plaques and healthy subjects exposed to naturally occurring asbestos. Lung. 2014;**192**(1):197-203

[71] Hu ZD, Liu XF, Liu XC, Ding CM, Hu CJ. Diagnostic accuracy of osteopontin for malignant pleural mesothelioma: A systematic review and meta-analysis. Clinica Chimica Acta. 2014;**433**:44-48

[72] Bruno F, Baratti D, Martinetti A, Morelli D, Sottotetti E, Bonini C, et al. Mesothelin and osteopontin as circulating markers of diffuse malignant peritoneal mesothelioma: A preliminary study. European Journal of Surgical Oncology. 2018;**44**(6):792-798

[73] Mastrangelo G, Marangi G, Ballarin MN, Michilin S, Fabricio AS, Valentini F, et al. Osteopontin, asbestos exposure and pleural plaques: A cross-sectional study. BMC Public Health. 2011;**11**:220

[74] Kovac V, Zwitter M, Zagar T. Improved survival after introduction of chemotherapy for malignant pleural mesothelioma in Slovenia: Population-based survey of 444 patients. Radiology and Oncology. 2012;**46**(2):136-144

[75] Johnen G, Gawrych K, Raiko I, Casjens S, Pesch B, Weber DG, et al. Calretinin as a blood-based biomarker for mesothelioma. BMC Cancer. 2017;**17**(1):386

[76] Husain AN, Colby TV, Ordonez NG, Allen TC, Attanoos RL, Beasley MB, et al. Guidelines for pathologic diagnosis

of malignant mesothelioma 2017 update of the consensus statement from the international mesothelioma interest group. Archives of Pathology & Laboratory Medicine. 2018;**142**(1):89-108

[77] Johnen G, Burek K, Raiko I, Wichert K, Pesch B, Weber DG, et al. Prediagnostic detection of mesothelioma by circulating calretinin and mesothelin - a case-control comparison nested into a prospective cohort of asbestos-exposed workers. Scientific Reports. 2018;**8**(1):14321

[78] Jiménez-Ramírez C, Casjens S, Juárez-Pérez CA, Raiko I, Del Razo LM, Taeger D, et al. Mesothelin, Calretinin, and Megakaryocyte Potentiating Factor as Biomarkers of Malignant Pleural Mesothelioma. 2019. DOI: 10.1007/s00408-019-00244-1. [Epub ahead of print]

[79] Raiko I, Sander I, Weber DG, Raulf-Heimsoth M, Gillissen A, Kollmeier J, et al. Development of an enzyme-linked immunosorbent assay for the detection of human calretinin in plasma and serum of mesothelioma patients. BMC Cancer. 2010;**10**:242

[80] Aguilar-Madrid G, Pesch B, Calderon-Aranda ES, Burek K, Jimenez-Ramirez C, Juarez-Perez CA, et al. Biomarkers for predicting malignant pleural mesothelioma in a Mexican population. International Journal of Medical Sciences. 2018;**15**(9):883-891

[81] Blum W, Schwaller B. Calretinin is essential for mesothelioma cell growth/survival in vitro: A potential new target for malignant mesothelioma therapy? International Journal of Cancer. 2013;**133**(9):2077-2088

[82] Worthmuller J, Blum W, Pecze L, Salicio V, Schwaller B. Calretinin promotes invasiveness and EMT in malignant mesothelioma cells involving the activation of the FAK signaling pathway. Oncotarget. 2018;**9**(91):36256-36272

[83] Creaney J, Robinson BWS. Malignant mesothelioma biomarkers: From discovery to use in clinical practice for diagnosis, monitoring, screening, and treatment. Chest. 2017;**152**(1):143-149

[84] Cristaudo A, Bonotti A, Guglielmi G, Fallahi P, Foddis R. Serum mesothelin and other biomarkers: What have we learned in the last decade? Journal of Thoracic Disease. 2018;**10**(Suppl 2):S353-S359

[85] Foddis R, Bonotti A, Landi S, Fallahi P, Guglielmi G, Cristaudo A. Biomarkers in the prevention and follow-up of workers exposed to asbestos. Journal of Thoracic Disease. 2018;**10**(Suppl 2):S360-S368

[86] Kirschner MB, Cheng YY, Badrian B, Kao SC, Creaney J, Edelman JJ, et al. Increased circulating miR-625-3p: A potential biomarker for patients with malignant pleural mesothelioma. Journal of Thoracic Oncology. 2012;7(7):1184-1191

[87] Micolucci L, Akhtar MM, Olivieri F, Rippo MR, Procopio AD. Diagnostic value of microRNAs in asbestos exposure and malignant mesothelioma: Systematic review and qualitative meta-analysis. Oncotarget. 2016;7(36):58606-58637

[88] Mozzoni P, Ampollini L, Goldoni M, Alinovi R, Tiseo M, Gnetti L, et al. MicroRNA expression in malignant pleural mesothelioma and asbestosis: A pilot study. Disease Markers. 2017;**2017**:9645940

[89] Santarelli L, Gaetani S, Monaco F, Bracci M, Valentino M, Amati M, et al. Four-miRNA signature to identify asbestos-related lung malignancies. Cancer Epidemiology, Biomarkers & Prevention. 2019;**28**(1):119-126

[90] Bonotti A, Simonini S, Pantani E, Giusti L, Donadio E, Mazzoni MR, et al. Serum mesothelin, osteopontin and vimentin: Useful markers for clinical monitoring of malignant pleural mesothelioma. The International Journal of Biological Markers. 2017;**32**(1):e126-e131

[91] Felten MK, Khatab K, Knoll L, Schettgen T, Muller-Berndorff H, Kraus T. Changes of mesothelin and osteopontin levels over time in formerly asbestos-exposed power industry workers. International Archives of Occupational and Environmental Health. 2014;**87**(2):195-204

[92] Battolla E, Canessa PA, Ferro P, Franceschini MC, Fontana V, Dessanti P, et al. Comparison of the diagnostic performance of Fibulin-3 and Mesothelin in patients with pleural effusions from malignant mesothelioma. Anticancer Research. 2017;**37**(3):1387-1391

Chapter 3

Asbestos Exposure Results in Asbestosis and Usual Interstitial Pneumonia Similar to Other Causes of Pneumoconiosis

Yoshinori Kawabata

Abstract

The progression of asbestosis is supposed to begin with the first order of respiratory bronchiole and extend outward. Recently, grade 4 asbestosis was reported to begin with the subpleural peripheral lobular area or the subpleural lobule. Grade 4 asbestosis is defined as diffuse pulmonary fibrosis caused by the inhalation of excessive numbers of asbestos fibers. Pathologically, the presence of more than two asbestos bodies/cm^2 on a glass slide is required. There are many cases of diffuse interstitial pneumonia, mainly usual interstitial pneumonia, that does not fulfill the above criteria among asbestos workers or high-grade environmentally exposed persons. I call these cases "usual interstitial pneumonia seen in asbestos workers" and not idiopathic pulmonary fibrosis. In this chapter, I discuss the above subjects, including the dose-response relationship for asbestos exposure, the heterogeneous response to asbestos exposure, and the relationship between asbestosis and idiopathic pulmonary fibrosis.

Keywords: pathological examination, usual interstitial pneumonia, atelectatic induration, asbestos body, idiopathic pulmonary fibrosis

1. Introduction

It is well known that moderate- to high-grade exposures to asbestos cause serious diffuse pulmonary fibrosis called diffuse asbestosis. Asbestosis is believed to start in the region of the first order of respiratory bronchiole (grade 1, **Figure 1**) and gradually extends outward to involve more and more of the lung acinus until separate foci of fibrosis link or attach to the pleura and the interlobular septum (grade 3), finally resulting in a diffuse pattern of the fibrosis (grade 4) [1, 2]. However, this description has not yet been proved. Asbestosis is defined as diffuse interstitial fibrosis of the lung as a consequence of exposure to asbestos dust. A histological diagnosis of asbestosis requires the presence of two or more asbestos bodies (ABs) in the tissue with a section area of 1 cm^2 [3]. Meanwhile, diffuse interstitial pneumonia, mainly usual interstitial pneumonia (UIP), that does not fulfill the above histological criteria is called idiopathic pulmonary fibrosis (IPF) even if the patient is a worker exposed to asbestos [4].

In this review, I discuss the process of asbestosis progression, the pathological definition and the features of asbestosis, the lower limit of asbestos fiber exposure

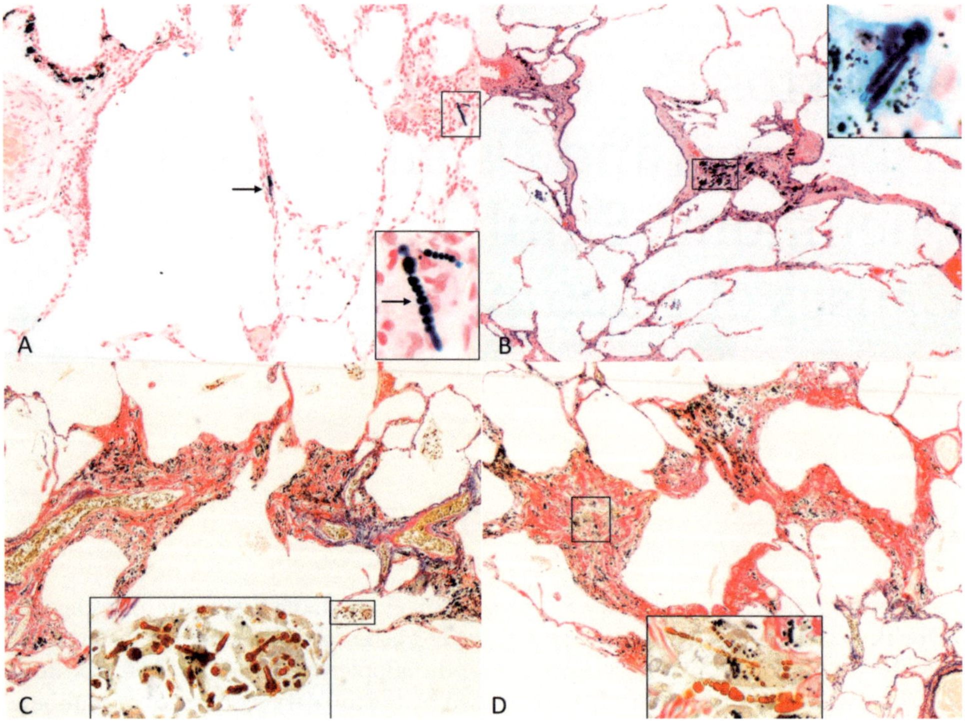

Figure 1.
Grade 0 to grade 2 lesions. (A) Grade 0 lesion without respiratory bronchiolar fibrosis but with three asbestos bodies (arrows). Hematoxylin and eosin staining (HE), ×100. Inset: enlarged asbestos bodies. (B) Grade 1 lesion with fibrosis of the respiratory bronchiole and surrounding lung. HE, ×60. Inset: enlarged asbestos bodies. (C) Grade 2 lesion with fibrosis of the respiratory bronchiole and surrounding lung. Elastica van Gieson staining (EvG), ×60. Inset: many enlarged asbestos bodies. (D) Grade 2 lesion with fibrosis of the respiratory bronchiole, alveolar duct, and surrounding lung including luminal organization. EvG, ×60. Inset: enlarged asbestos bodies.

causing asbestosis and the dose-response relationship of asbestos exposure, various causes of UIP, and how to think about diffuse interstitial pneumonia or UIP that does not fulfill the histological criteria of asbestosis. The term "asbestosis" is used differently in the literature. I term diffuse interstitial fibrosis due to asbestos exposure as pathological grade 4 asbestosis and clinical diffuse asbestosis. The term asbestosis alone can indicate various extents of severity from grade 1 to grade 4 pathologically and early to diffuse asbestosis clinically.

2. Process of asbestosis progression

Under a normal environmental state, the numbers of ABs are thought to be up to 200 per gram of dry lung tissue (/g dry lung) [5, 6], and the presence of more than 1000 ABs/g dry lung is thought to indicate persons with a high probability of exposure to asbestos dust at work [3, 7]. As stated above, asbestosis begins in the first order of respiratory bronchiole (**Figure 1**), but how many ABs are needed to cause grade 1 asbestosis? The minimal numbers are different from study to study and range from "1,000 to 22,000" ABs/g dry lung [5, 6, 8–10]. Our data showed a maximum of "273,000" ABs/g dry lung in grade 4 asbestosis without grade 1 lesions [9], and this might be the upper limit. Meanwhile, there are reports showing the presence of grade 1 fibrosis of below 1 AB per 1 histological slide even in cases of diffuse asbestosis [11, 12]. Grade 1 lesions appear to begin at lowest numbers of less than 1000 ABs/g dry lung, but the upper limit is not precisely known yet except for that in our data [9]. Thus, it is still necessary to determine how many ABs or asbestos fibers are needed to cause grade 1 and grade 2 lesions without progression to grade 4 asbestosis.

Meanwhile, one of the important pathological criteria of idiopathic UIP (IPF) is predominant subpleural and/or paraseptal distribution of fibrosis mainly in the lower lobes [13, 14]. This means that UIP begins in a peripheral area of the lobule with continuous extension inward and forms centrilobular honeycombing due to peripheral lobular dense fibrosis and structural destruction of the centrilobular area. An outward extension of asbestosis to form centrilobular honeycombing of grade 4 asbestosis is a logical contradiction. It might be logical to think that grade 4 asbestosis is not just a further outward extension of grade 3 asbestosis. We examined grade 4 asbestosis histologically and confirmed that UIP-type asbestosis begins with the subpleural peripheral lobular area as this area was the most densely fibrotic (intraluminal collagenosis with collapse) and the centrilobular area showed young fibrosis (**Figure 2**) including fibroblastic foci. We also observed inflammatory cell infiltration and lymphoid follicles in the fibrosis-like idiopathic UIP [9]. We also confirmed that atelectatic induration-type asbestosis also begins with the subpleural peripheral lobular area or the subpleural lobule (acinar or lobular intraluminal collagenosis with various degrees of collapse with inflammatory cell infiltration) (**Figure 3**) [9]. Yamamoto also stated nearly the same in terms of the starting point of grade 4 asbestosis [11]. Inflammatory cell infiltration was reported in humans [15, 16] and experimental sheep along with intraluminal organization [17].

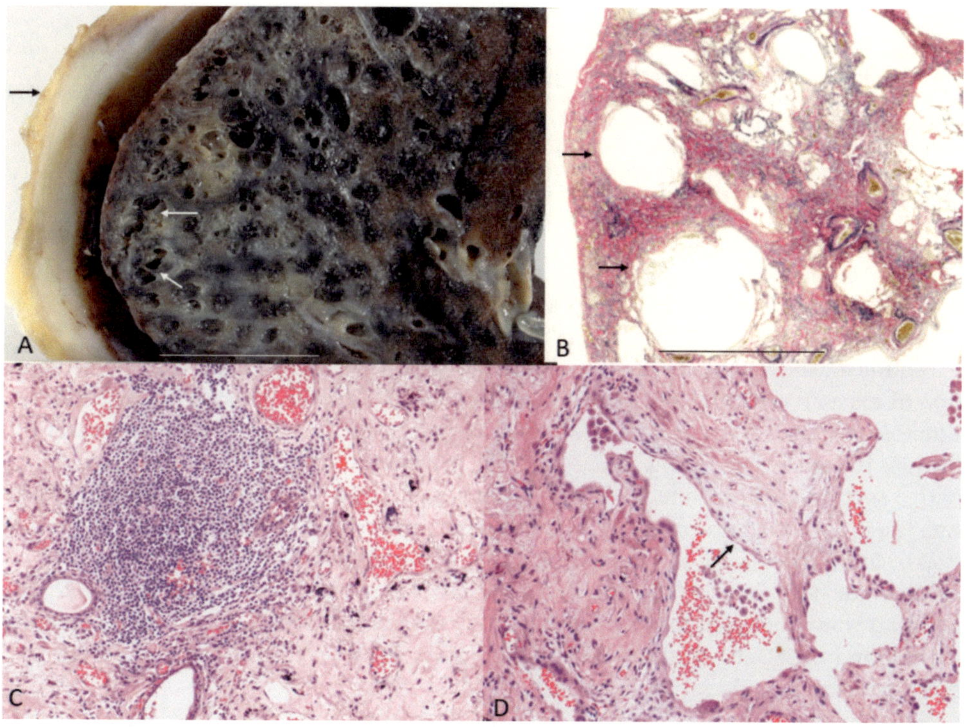

Figure 2.
Histology of usual interstitial pneumonia-type asbestosis in a 66-year-old man working with rock wool spray. A lobectomy was performed for lung cancer. Upon examination, the numbers of asbestos bodies (ABs) were 950,000 ABs/g dry lung and 108 ABs/cm². A grade 2 lesion was seen (Figure 1C, D). Macroscopic features of the right lower lobe showed diffuse formation of pleural plaques (black arrow) and honeycombing (white arrows) in the gray-colored fibrosis of the lung. Bar = 2 cm. Histological features showed subpleural dense fibrosis with ring-like honeycombing (arrow). Elastica van Gieson, ×10. Bar = 5 mm. One lymphoid follicle was noted in the fibrosis. Hematoxylin and eosin (HE), ×150. Young intraluminal fibrosis was noted between dense fibrosis and the normal lung. HE, ×150.

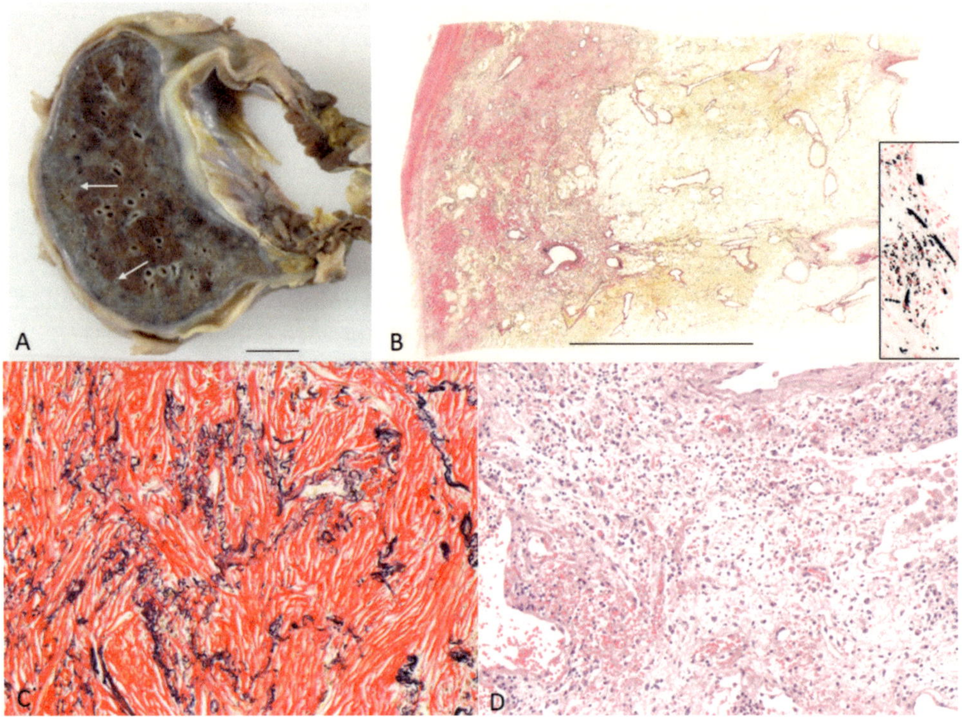

Figure 3.
Atelectatic induration-type asbestosis in a 60-year-old man working in the asbestos cement industry for 30 years as a secretary. Bilateral diffuse pleural thickening with calcification and reticular shadows in the bilateral basal areas of the lower lobes. No grade 1 lesion was seen. (A) Macroscopic features of the right lower lobe showed pleural fibrosis and plaque at the diaphragmatic area with subpleural zonal atelectatic induration (arrow). Bar = 2.5 cm. (B) Panoramic view of the subpleural lung tissue showing 1-cm-thick subpleural atelectatic induration. Hematoxylin and eosin. Bar = 1 cm. Inset. Asbestos bodies stained with Persian blue. (C) Subpleural area showing intraluminal dense fibrosis and muscle proliferation with some collapse. Elastica van Gieson, ×200. (D) Young intraluminal fibrosis with inflammatory cell infiltration next to normal lung.

3. Pathological definition of grade 4 asbestosis and its features

Grade 4 asbestosis is defined as diffuse pulmonary fibrosis caused by the inhalation of excessive numbers of asbestos fibers [1–3, 7]. The Helsinki criteria state that a histological diagnosis of asbestosis requires the identification of diffuse interstitial fibrosis in well-inflated lung tissue plus the presence of two or more ABs in tissue with a section area of 1 cm^2 [3, 7]. The previous histological definition of asbestosis was the presence of one or more ABs in one or another histological section in addition to lung fibrosis [1]. A subsequent study showed that more ABs are needed to cause grade 4 asbestosis [18]. Then, more than 2 ABs/cm^2 were required in 1997 [3], and that was continued in the next Helsinki criteria [7]. Two ABs/cm^2 on glass slides correspond to "8000–20,000" ABs or over/g dry lung [12, 19, 20]. The smallest numbers were less than "4000" ABs in our data [9].

Histological findings of grade 4 asbestosis show various forms: atelectatic induration type or accelerated asbestosis and UIP pattern (**Figures 2** and **3**) [2, 9, 11]. I described the histological features of atelectatic induration and UIP pattern in the previous chapter. The asbestos burden in atelectatic induration is more severe than that in the UIP pattern [9]. It is reported that atelectatic induration type is seen in undeveloped countries, and UIP is seen in developed countries [2]. It is also reported that fibrosis in asbestosis is always paucicellular, lacks any significant degree of inflammation, and is collagenous rather than fibroblastic, without reference to other studies [2]. From this viewpoint, Kishimoto et al. reported the mean value of ABs for these cases was a mean of "2,133,000"/g dry lung [21], whereas Arakawa et al. reported a mean of "1,465,000" [22]. However, it is difficult to point out specific histological features seen only in asbestosis [3, 7, 9, 11, 23]. Yamamoto stated that some cases cannot be differentiated from that of IPF except for the presence of ABs [11]. Patterns of fibrosing nonspecific interstitial pneumonia and unclassifiable interstitial pneumonia were also reported [2, 22, 24].

What asbestos burden is required to cause grade 4 asbestosis? We reported it to be between "3,450 and 3,340,000" ABs/g dry lung [9], and Kishimoto et al. reported a value between "156,000 and 2,733,000" ABs [21]. Arakawa et al. reported a mean of "1,465,000" [22] with the highest number being "7,473,000" ABs (personal communication). Roggli et al. have reported the highest numbers, which range from "6,840,000 to 16,000,000" ABs/g dry lung [5, 8]. So, as with the beginning of grade 1 asbestosis, there are enormous differences from person to person in the number of ABs that indicate grade 4 asbestosis.

Chrysotile fibers (one of commercially produced and most used asbestos fibers) are difficult to coat with iron (during AB formation) and are easily dissolved and cleared from the lung [25, 26]. There are reports of asbestosis without ABs histologically but which show numerous asbestos fibers in the lung [27, 28]. In cases of asbestos exposure with diffuse pulmonary fibrosis that do not fulfill the Helsinki criteria, it is then necessary to determine the numbers of asbestos fibers in the lung using electron microscopy. Still, this may not be enough as most chrysotile fibers are cleared by the time of examination [25, 26], but long chrysotile fibers can become asbestos body [29].

4. Lower limit of asbestos fiber exposure causing asbestosis and the dose-response relationship

For clinical purposes, the following guidelines are recommended to identify persons with a high probability of exposure to asbestos dust: over "0.1 million" amphibole fibers (>5 μm)/g dry lung tissue, over "1 million" amphibole fibers (>1 μm)/g dry lung tissue as measured by electron microscopy in a qualified laboratory, or over "1000" ABs/g dry lung tissue, among others [3, 7]. The relationship between asbestos exposure and disease onset or early asbestosis is not settled yet. Precise estimation of the cumulative exposure amount is difficult and may actually be impossible.

It is reported that clinical asbestosis can be induced by cumulative asbestos exposure to around 25 to 200 fibers/mL-years [2, 23, 30–32]. However, there are many reports concerning the beginning of asbestosis. Green et al. reported that asbestosis was usually present in asbestos textile workers exposed to more than 20 fibers/mL-years [33]. Fischer et al. reported 42% of patients with asbestosis do not reach an exposure level of 25 fibers/mL-years [10]. The smallest exposure causing early asbestosis radiologically or histologically might be less than 2–5 fibers/mL-years [34–36]. Fischer et al. also reported that the clinical estimate of fibers/mL-years does not correlate with the numbers of ABs/g dry lung and the beginning of grade 1 lesions [10]. One reason might be differences in the ability to decompose or detoxify the inhaled asbestos fibers from person to person. Another reason is that chrysotile is easily cleared from the lung and is difficult to coat with iron as stated earlier [23, 24]. The development and progression of asbestosis are generally independently correlated with cumulative asbestos exposure and latency, and the dose–response curve is nonlinear [32, 37–45]. Heavy exposure shortens latency, and diffuse asbestosis has been reported with 13 years of latency [46, 47]. In contrast, new lesions appear at a mean of 35 years of latency [48], and there is one report of rapidly progressive pulmonary interstitial fibrosis appearing with 40 years of latency [49].

Even a high level of environmental exposure (living near asbestos mines or asbestos factories, families of asbestos workers, and others) can result in mild or early asbestosis (either grade 1 or 2 lesions or early UIP-type fibrosis) [50–55]. From these previous studies [50–55], it is not clear whether such a level of exposure causes grade 4 asbestosis or diffuse UIP-type fibrosis.

As stated above, an exposure level of 20–25 fibers/mL-years is supposed to indicate the beginning of asbestosis, but actually a lower level of 2 fibers/mL-years can cause early asbestosis or early UIP-type fibrosis based on long-term follow-up. The main reason for the variable response to exposure might be the different abilities of humans to digest, clear, transport, and detoxify asbestos fibers, and thus their susceptibility can differ [56]. In addition genetic polymorphisms affect the fibrogenesis and carcinogenesis of asbestos fibers [57–60].

The beginning of grade 1 lesions occurs between "1,000 and 273,000" ABs/g dry lung, whereas grade 4 asbestosis satisfying the Helsinki Criteria is between "3,450 and 16,000,000" ABs/g dry lung. The dose-response relationship has been determined, but small numbers of people do not have asbestosis even when they suffered from near the upper limits of exposure. The essential question is whether there is a threshold asbestos dose that causes pulmonary fibrosis.

5. Relationship between IPF and asbestos exposure

Gaensler et al. reported a 5% incidence of IPF in workers exposed to asbestos [4]. This incidence is higher than that of 0.002% among American people 75 years or older [61]. Roggli et al. reported the mean ABs/g dry lung in IPF cases to be 90 (8–1480)/g dry lung, whereas it was 30 (2–220) in normal people [5]. We reported that asbestos exposure increases the incidence of UIP [62]. Barber et al. reported that for mesothelioma and IPF, there was a significant linear relationship between the number of male and female deaths each year and historic imports of asbestos in the UK, and for mortality from asbestosis, a similar relationship was found for male but not female deaths [63, 64]. They selected a latent period of 48 years based on a previously developed US asbestosis model [65]. Attanoos et al. also reported the presence of three cases of UIP without ABs among asbestos workers [24]. We need to reconsider that mild to moderate amounts of asbestos exposure might cause diffuse UIP. A schematic relationship between asbestos exposure and diffuse pulmonary fibrosis is presented in **Figure 4**. It might be more appropriate not to call IPF that does not fulfill the Helsinki Criteria but results from more than environmental exposure or low-grade occupational exposure level "diffuse pulmonary fibrosis or UIP seen in asbestos exposed person."

Figure 5 illustrates such a case of short-term occupational exposure occurring more than 40 years ago that was followed up as IPF. Macroscopic and microscopic features are identical with those of IPF. Most of the analyzed asbestos fibers were chrysotile with not enough AB formation to call it asbestosis [66].

Many epidemiologic studies have reported the risk factors of IPF as being male, smoking, having a specific occupation (with exposure to wood dust, metal dust, sand/silica, mining, engineering, agriculture, animal dust, and others), or hobby (raising birds and others) [67–73]. These data suggest that IPF can be triggered by various inciting agents in genetically susceptible persons. Investigation into genetic risk factors such as telomere length and the *Muc5B* rs35705950 promoter polymorphism is now underway [74–78].

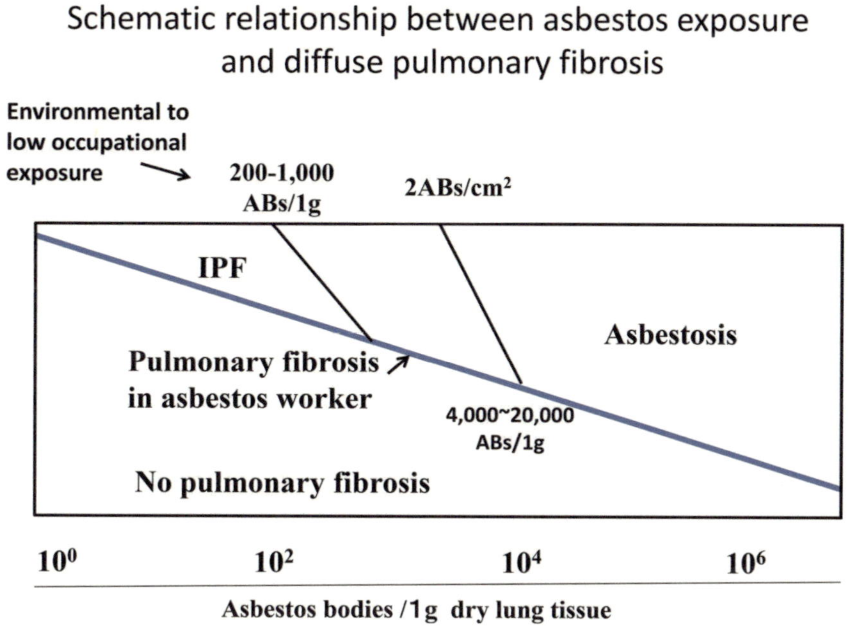

Figure 4.
Schematic of the suspected relationship between asbestos exposure and diffuse pulmonary fibrosis. By increasing asbestos exposure, the frequency of diffuse pulmonary fibrosis increases proportionately. When more than 2 asbestos bodies (ABs)/cm² are found histologically, this fibrosis can be termed asbestosis. When ABs in the digested lung are present between environmental and low occupational levels (200–1000 ABs/g) and less than 2 ABs/cm², this fibrosis can be termed idiopathic pulmonary fibrosis (IPF) when no cause is found. The boundary between asbestosis and IPF can be called "pulmonary fibrosis in asbestos workers."

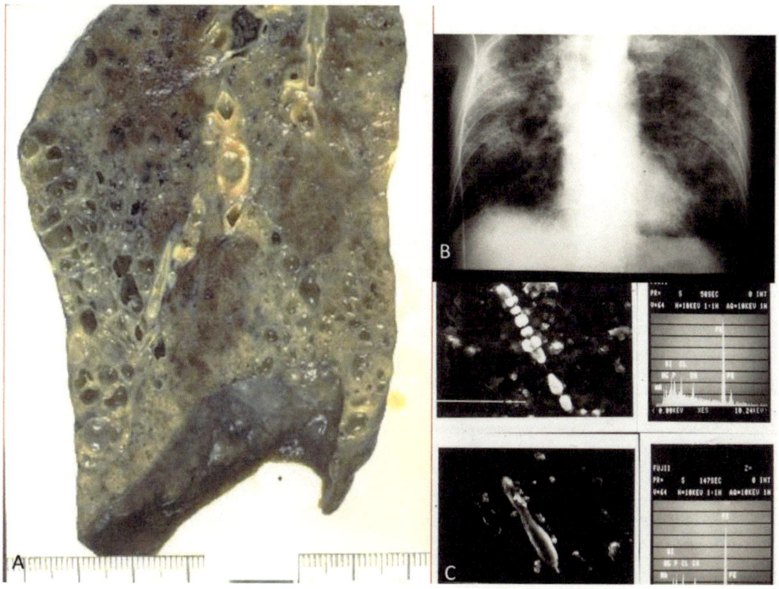

Figure 5.
Radiological and pathological features of an asbestos exposed worker that does not fulfill asbestosis criteria. A case of pulmonary fibrosis in a 73-year-old male asbestos worker who visited a hospital because of acutely progressive dyspnea. Clinically, this case was diagnosed as acute exacerbation of IPF. Usual interstitial pneumonia (UIP)-type fibrosis and pleural and pericardial plaques were found at autopsy. He had worked several months at a shipyard 40 years ago during war time. The number of asbestos bodies (ABs) was 740/g dry lung. Macroscopic features are typical for UIP with clear subpleural honeycombing in the right lower lobe, and no pleural fibrosis or adhesions were found. Plain chest X-ray showed diffuse infiltrative pulmonary shadows bilaterally. Typical (upper left) and atypical ABs (lower left) were found, but these were almost all composed of chrysotile as confirmed by energy-dispersive X-ray analysis (right).

6. UIP seen in various diseases

Various diseases cause UIP including various pneumoconioses, chronic hypersensitivity pneumonitis, and collagen vascular diseases. Histological features of pneumoconiosis are characterized by bronchiolocentric fibrous nodule formation predominantly in the upper lobes. Arakawa et al. reported a prevalence of chronic interstitial pneumonia in 243 pneumoconiosis cases of approximately 12% on CT, and three fourths of these cases showed a typical IPF pattern. Pathological data obtained by autopsy or lobectomy in 11 cases indicated UIP [79]. The prevalence of chronic interstitial pneumonia among pneumoconiosis cases is 10–20% [80–82]. Arakawa et al. reported that the earliest CT abnormalities (faint ground-glass opacity or coarse reticular opacity) of 14 cases appeared at the lung bases and then fibrosis progressed to honeycombing over a median period of 12.1 years in the silica-exposed patients, with autopsy in 8 cases confirming a diagnosis of typical UIP [83]. Generally, latent periods from occupational exposure to disease onset are quite long [79–83]. Occasionally, hard metal lung disease appears as UIP when the degree of exposure has been mild [84]. Histological features of acute and subacute hypersensitivity pneumonitis are characterized by bronchiolo-alveolitis with loose granulomas diffusely spread throughout both lungs. In contrast, most chronic hypersensitivity pneumonitis shows UIP pathologically, with points of differentiation from that of IPF being the presence of bronchiolitis, peribronchiolar fibrosis

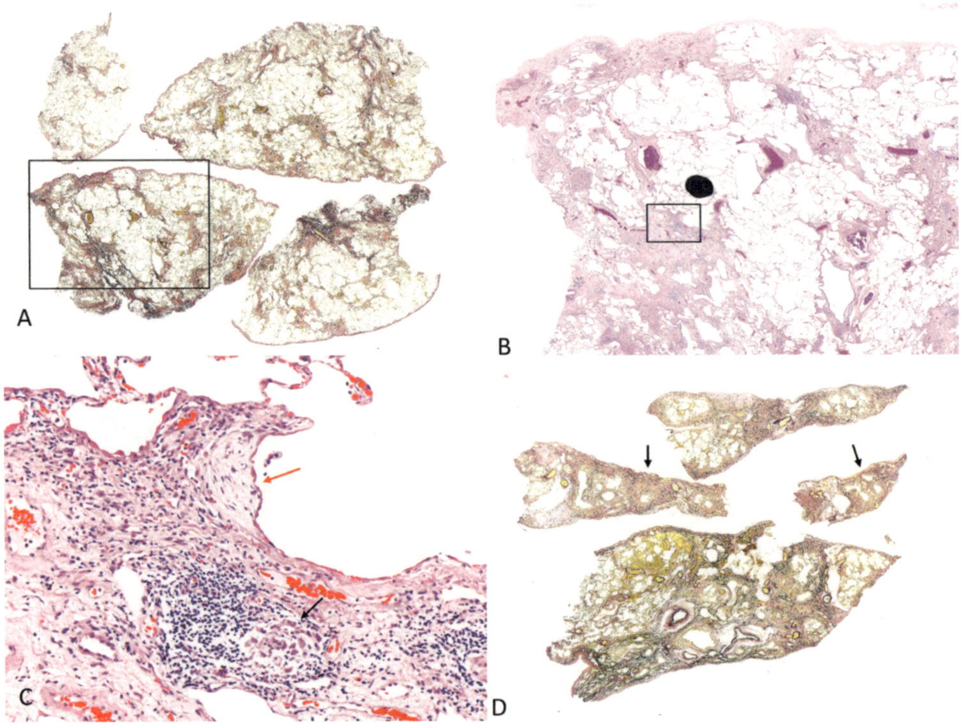

Figure 6.
Histology of chronic hypersensitivity pneumonia. A 66-year-old woman who had been breeding birds developed progressive dyspnea. Specific antigen for pigeon was markedly elevated. Surgical lung biopsy was performed from the left lingula and S8 (case from the Department of Respiratory Medicine, Kobe City Medical Center West Hospital). A panoramic view of the lingula showed mainly subpleural dense fibrosis. Elastica van Gieson staining (EvG). Patchy dense fibrosis was noted mainly in the subpleural area and peripheral lobular areas (next to an interlobular septum by EvG) of the lung. Box in A: hematoxylin and eosin (HE), ×40. A clear fibroblastic focus was noted at the edge of the dense fibrosis (red arrow), and one loose granuloma was seen in the fibrosis (black arrow). Box in B: HE, ×200. Panoramic view of the S8 showing subpleural dense fibrosis and honeycombing (black arrow). EvG.

or centrilobular fibrosis, bridging fibrosis, epithelioid cell granuloma, and giant cells [85–87]. Still, it is impossible to think of UIP as an extension of respiratory bronchiolar lesions as UIP begins within the subpleural peripheral lung. Typical histological features of chronic hypersensitivity pneumonitis are shown in **Figure 6**. Recently, telomere-related gene variants were reported in chronic hypersensitivity pneumonitis [88]. UIP is the one of the major pulmonary complications in cases of collagen vascular diseases, especially in rheumatoid arthritis (RA). As with IPF, the prevalence is higher in smokers and males [89]. UIP in RA shares a number of radiological and histopathological features with IPF [90–92]. An additional histological feature of UIP in RA is frequent germinal center formation [93]. RA-related UIP also begins within basal, subpleural peripheral areas as does IPF. Recently, the *MUC5B* promoter variant was reported in RA-related UIP [94].

7. Conclusion

Moderate to severe exposure to asbestos causes asbestosis. However, there are a number of cases of UIP in asbestos workers or high-grade environmentally exposed people that do not fulfill the Helsinki criteria. The susceptibility to asbestos exposure varies. UIP-type grade 4 asbestosis begins within the basal, subpleural peripheral areas as do cases of IPF, other pneumoconioses, chronic hypersensitivity pneumonitis, and RA. The suspected relationship between asbestos exposure, numbers of exposed persons, and the development of diffuse pulmonary fibrosis is shown in **Figure 7**. Cases of diffuse UIP with less than 200–1000 ABs/g dry lung

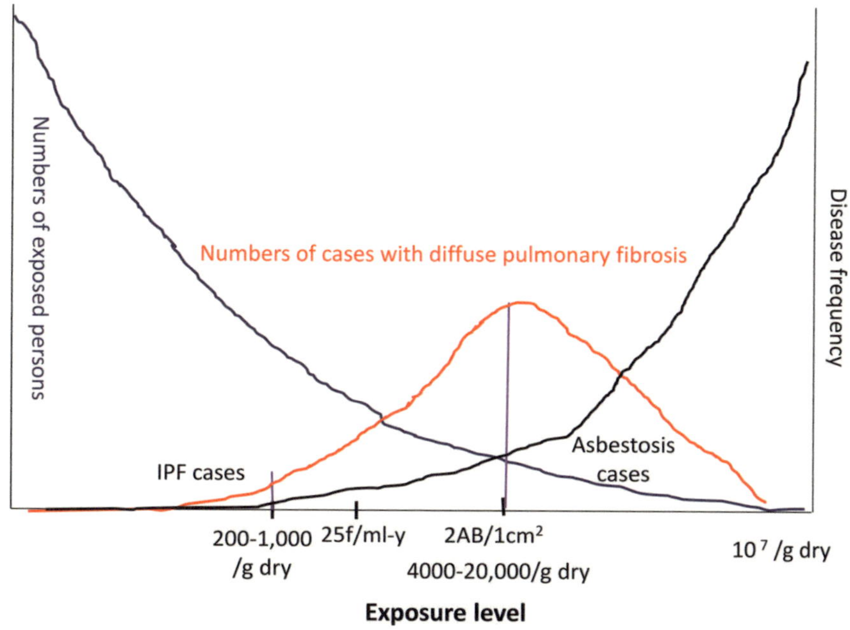

Figure 7.
Schematic of suspected cases of diffuse pulmonary fibrosis related to asbestos exposure. The black line is the suspected dose-response curve related to the degree of asbestos exposure and disease frequency. The lower line indicates the degree of asbestos exposure, with 200–100/g dry lung indicating higher than the environmental or low occupational exposure level, 25 f/mL-y indicating the beginning of the asbestosis level, and 2 asbestos bodies/cm² or 4000–20,000/g dry lung indicating the beginning of the grade 4 asbestosis exposure level. The blue line indicates the numbers of people exposed. The red line indicates the numbers of diffuse pulmonary fibrosis. Disease in patients with less than the low occupational level can be called idiopathic pulmonary fibrosis, whereas that in patients between the low occupational exposure level and grade 4 asbestosis exposure level can be called diffuse usual interstitial pneumonia seen in asbestos workers (or a high-grade environmentally exposed person).

can be called IPF when there is no other etiology. Diffuse interstitial fibrosis with more than 2 ABs/cm^2 can be called grade 4 asbestosis. There might be significant numbers of cases of diffuse interstitial fibrosis that lie between IPF and grade 4 asbestosis, and these cases can be called diffuse interstitial pneumonia seen in asbestos workers or high-grade environmentally exposed persons.

I hope future more genetic research can reveal the phenotypes that can acquire diffuse pulmonary fibrosis through mild occupational and environmental exposure to dust.

Acknowledgements

I am grateful to Prof. Andrew Churg (Department of Pathology, University of British Columbia, Vancouver, Canada) for his critical comments.

Conflict of interest

The author declares no conflicts of interest and no funding disclosures.

Author details

Yoshinori Kawabata
Division of Diagnostic Pathology, Saitama Prefectural Cardiovascular and Respiratory Center, Kumagaya, Japan

*Address all correspondence to: kawabata.yoshinori@pref.saitama.lg.jp

References

[1] Craighead JE, Abraham JL, Churg A, et al. The pathology of asbestos associated diseases of the lungs and pleural cavities: Diagnostic criteria and proposed grading schema (Report of the Pneumoconiosis Committee of the College of American Pathologists and the National Institute for Occupational Safety and Health). Archives of Pathology & Laboratory Medicine. 1982;**106**:544-596

[2] Roggli VL, Gibbs AR, Attanoos R, et al. Pathology of asbestosis- An update of the diagnostic criteria: Report of the asbestosis committee of the college of American pathologists and pulmonary pathology society. Archives of Pathology & Laboratory Medicine. 2010;**134**:462-480. DOI: 10.5858/arpa.2015-0503-SA

[3] Henderson DW, Rantanen J, Barnhart S, et al. Asbestos, asbestosis, and cancer: The Helsinki criteria for diagnosis and attribution. A consensus report of an international expert group. Scandinavian Journal of Work, Environment & Health. 1997;**28**:311-316

[4] Gaensler EA, Jederlinic PJ, Churg A. Idiopathic pulmonary fibrosis in asbestos-exposed workers. The American Review of Respiratory Disease. 1991;**144**:689-696

[5] Roggli VL, Pratt PC, Brody AR. Asbestos content of lung tissue in asbestos associated diseases: A study of 110 cases. British Journal of Industrial Medicine. 1986;**43**:18-28

[6] Kobayashi H, Watanabe H, Zhang WM, Ohnishi Y. A quantitative and histological study on pulmonary effects of asbestos exposure in general autopsied lungs. Acta Pathologica Japonica. 1986;**36**:1781-1791

[7] Wolff H, Vehmas T, Oksa P, Rantanen J, Vainio H. Asbestos, asbestosis, and cancer, the Helsinki criteria for diagnosis and attribution 2014: Recommendations. Scandinavian Journal of Work, Environment & Health. 2015;**41**:5-15. DOI: 10.5271/sjweh.3462

[8] Roggli VL, Vollmer RT. Twenty-five years of fiber analysis: What have we learned? Human Pathology. 2008;**39**:307-315. DOI: 10.1016/j.humpath.2007.07.005

[9] Kawabata Y, Kasai T, Kobashi Y, et al. Grade 4 asbestosis does not extend directly from the respiratory bronchiole to the peripheral lung. Histopathology. 2018;**73**:29-37. DOI: 10.1111/his.13493

[10] Fischer M, Gunther S, Muller KM. Fibre-years, pulmonary asbestos burden and asbestosis. International Journal of Hygiene and Environmental Health. 2002;**205**:245-248

[11] Yamamoto S. Histopathological features of pulmonary asbestosis with particular emphasis on the comparison with those of usual interstitial pneumonia. Osaka City Medical Journal. 1997;**43**:225-242

[12] Warnock ML, Wolery G. Asbestos bodies or fibres and the diagnosis of asbestosis. Environmental Research. 1987;**44**:29-44

[13] Lynch DA, Sverzellati N, Travis WD, et al. Diagnostic criteria for idiopathic pulmonary fibrosis: A Fleischner Society White Paper. The Lancet Respiratory Medicine. 2018;**6**:138-153. DOI: 10.1016/S2213-2600(17)30433-2

[14] Raghu G, Remy-Jardi M, Myers JL, et al. Diagnosis of idiopathic pulmonary fibrosis an official ATS/ERS/JRS/ALAT clinical practice guideline. American Journal of Respiratory and Critical Care Medicine. 2018;**198**:e44-e68. DOI: 10.1164/rccm.201807-1255ST

[15] McDonald S. Histology of pulmonary asbestosis. British Medical Journal. 1927;**2**:1025-1026

[16] Sporn TA, Roggli VL. Asbestosis. In: Roggli VL, Oury TD, Sporn TA, editors. Pathology of Asbestos-Associated Diseases. 2nd ed. New York: Springer; 2004. pp. 71-103

[17] Sébastien P, Bégin R, Masse S. Mass, number and size of lung fibres in the pathogenesis of asbestosis in sheep. Journal of Experimental Pathology (Oxford, England). 1990;**71**:1-10

[18] Roggli VL, Pratt PC, Brody AR. Analysis of tissue mineral fiber content. In: Roggli VL, Greenberg SD, Pratt PC, editors. Pathology of Asbestos-Associated Diseases. Boston, MA: Little, Brown & Co Inc.; 1992. pp. 299-345

[19] Hiroshima K. Report to the Ministry of the Environment of Japan 2012. Pathological and Radiographic Evaluation of Asbestos Exposure. Tokyo Women's Medical University; 2012

[20] Roggli VL, Pratt PC. Numbers of asbestos bodies on iron-stained tissue sections in relation to asbestos body counts in lung tissue digests. Human Pathology. 1983;**14**:355-361

[21] Kishimoto T, Kato K, Arakawa H, Ashizawa K, Inai K, Takeshima Y. Clinical, radiological, and pathological investigation of asbestosis. International Journal of Environmental Research and Public Health. 2011;**8**:899-912. DOI: 10.3390/ijerph8030899

[22] Arakawa H, Kishimoto T, Ashizawa K, et al. Asbestosis and other pulmonary fibrosis in asbestos-exposed workers: High-resolution CT features with pathological correlations. European Radiology. 2016;**26**:1485-1492. DOI: 10.1007/s00330-015-3973-z

[23] Churg A. Nonneoplastic disease caused by asbestos. In: Churg A, Green FHY, editors. Pathology of Occupational Lung Disease. 2nd ed. Baltimore, MD: Williams & Wilkins; 1998. pp. 277-338

[24] Attanoos RL, Alchami FS, Pooley FD, Gibbs AR. Usual interstitial pneumonia in asbestos-exposed cohorts - concurrent idiopathic pulmonary fibrosis or atypical asbestosis? Histopathology. 2016;**69**: 492-498. DOI: 10.1111/his.12951

[25] Churg A. Deposition and clearance of chrysotile asbestos. The Annals of Occupational Hygiene. 1994;**38**:625-633, 424-425

[26] Churg A, Wright JL, Gilks B, DePaoli L. Rapid short-term clearance of chrysotile compared with amosite asbestos in the guinea pig. The American Review of Respiratory Disease. 1989;**139**:885-890

[27] Miller A, Langer AM, Teirstein AS, Selikoff IJ. "Nonspecific" interstitial pulmonary fibrosis. Association with asbestos fibers detected by electron microscopy. The New England Journal of Medicine. 1975;**292**:91-93

[28] Monsó E, Tura JM, Pujadas J, Morell F, Ruiz J, Morera J. Lung dust content in idiopathic pulmonary fibrosis: A study with scanning electron microscopy and energy dispersive x ray analysis. British Journal of Industrial Medicine. 1991;**48**:327-331

[29] Holden J, Churg A. Asbestos bodies and the diagnosis of asbestosis in chrysotile workers. Environmental Research. 1986;**39**:232-236

[30] Dupres JS, Mustard JF, Uffen RJ. Report of the Royal Commission on Matters of Health and Safety Arising From the Use of Asbestos in Ontario. Queen's Printer for Ontario: Toronto, Canada; 1984

[31] De Vuyst P, Gevenois PA. Asbestosis. In: Hendrick DJ, Burge PS, Beckett WS,

Churg A, editors. Occupational Disorders of the Lung: Recognition, Management, and Prevention. London: Saunders; 2002. pp. 143-162

[32] Browne K. A threshold for asbestos-related lung cancer. British Journal of Industrial Medicine. 1986;**43**:556-558

[33] Green FH, Harley R, Vallyathan V, et al. Exposure and mineralogical correlates of pulmonary fibrosis in chrysotile asbestos workers. Occupational and Environmental Medicine. 1997;**54**:549-559

[34] Sluis-Cremer GK. Asbestos disease at low exposure after long residence time in amphibole miners. Toxicology and Industrial Health. 1991;7:89-95

[35] Sluis-Cremer GK, Hnizdo E, du Toit RS. Evidence for an amphibole asbestos threshold exposure for asbestosis assessed by autopsy in South African asbestos miners. The Annals of Occupational Hygiene. 1990;**34**:443-451

[36] Johansson LG, Albin MP, Jakobsson KM, Welinder HE, Ranstam PJ, Attewell RG. Ferruginous bodies and pulmonary fibrosis in dead low to moderately exposed asbestos cement workers: Histological examination. British Journal of Industrial Medicine. 1987;**44**:550-558

[37] Berry G, Gilson JC, Holmes S, Lewinsohn H, Roach S. Asbestosis: A study of dose response relationships in an asbestos textile factory. British Journal of Industrial Medicine. 1979;**36**:98-112

[38] Finkelstein MM. Asbestosis in long-term employees of an Ontario asbestos-cement factory. The American Review of Respiratory Disease. 1982;**125**:496-501

[39] Lockey JE, Brooks SM, Jarabek AM, et al. Pulmonary changes after exposure to vermiculite contaminated with fibrous tremolite. The American Review of Respiratory Disease. 1984;**129**:952-958

[40] Ehrlich R, Lilis R, Chan E, Nicholson WJ, Selikoff IJ. Long term radiological effects of short term exposure to amosite asbestos among factory workers. British Journal of Industrial Medicine. 1992;**49**:268-275

[41] Jakobsson K, Strömberg U, Albin M, Welinder H, Hagmar L. Radiological changes in asbestos cement workers. Occupational and Environmental Medicine. 1995;**52**:20-27

[42] Stayner LT, Smith R, Bailer J, et al. Exposure-response analysis of respiratory disease risk associated with occupational exposure to chrysotile asbestos. Occupational and Environmental Medicine. 1997;**54**:646-652

[43] Paris C, Benichou J, Raffaelli C, et al. Factors associated with early-stage pulmonary fibrosis as determined by high-resolution computed tomography among persons occupationally exposed to asbestos. Scandinavian Journal of Work, Environment & Health. 2004;**30**:206-214

[44] Paris C, Martin A, Letourneux M, Wild P. Modelling prevalence and incidence of fibrosis and pleural plaques in asbestos-exposed populations for screening and follow-up: A cross-sectional study. Environmental Health. 2008;7:30. DOI: 10.1186/1476-069X-7-30

[45] Deng Q, Wang X, Wang M, Lan Y. Exposure-response relationship between chrysotile exposure and mortality from lung cancer and asbestosis. Occupational and Environmental Medicine. 2012;**69**: 81-86. DOI: 10.1136/oem.2011.064899

[46] Merewether ERA, Price GW. Report on Effects of Asbestos Dust on the Lungs and Suppression in the Asbestos

Industry. London: Her Majesty's Stationery Office; 1930. pp. 5-31

[47] Goff AM, Gaensler EA. Asbestosis following brief exposure in cigarette filter manufacture. Respiration. 1972;**29**:83-93

[48] Becklake MR, Liddell FD, Manfreda J, McDonald JC. Radiological changes after withdrawal from asbestos exposure. British Journal of Industrial Medicine. 1979;**36**:23-28

[49] Moy EV, Hu H, Christiani DC. A retired shipyard worker with rapidly progressive pulmonary interstitial fibrosis. Environmental Health Perspectives. 1999;**107**:321-327

[50] Kilburn KH, Lilis R, Anderson HA, et al. Asbestos diseases in family contacts of shipyard workers. American Journal of Public Health. 1985;**75**:615-617

[51] Magnani C, Mollo F, Paoletti L, et al. Asbestos lung burden and asbestosis after occupational and environmental exposure in an asbestos cement manufacturing area: A necropsy study. Occupational and Environmental Medicine. 1998;**55**:840-846

[52] Hilbert TJ, Franzblau A, Dunning KK, Borton EK, Rohs AM, Lockey JE. Asbestos-related radiographic findings among household contacts of workers exposed to Libby vermiculite: Impact of workers' personal hygiene practices. Journal of Occupational and Environmental Medicine. 2013;**55**:1300-1304. DOI: 10.1097/JOM.0b013e31829fcf1a

[53] Lee EK, Kim JS, Kim Y, Park JS. CT findings in people who were environmentally exposed to asbestos in Korea. Journal of Korean Medical Science. 2015;**30**:1896-1901. DOI: 10.3346/jkms.2015.30.12.1896

[54] Kim Y, Myong JP, Lee JK, Kim JS, Kim YK, Jung SH. CT characteristics of pleural plaques related to occupational or environmental asbestos exposure from South Korean asbestos mines. Korean Journal of Radiology. 2015;**16**:1142-1152. DOI: 10.3348/kjr.2015.16.5.1142

[55] Kang D, Kim YY, Shin M, et al. Relationships of lower lung fibrosis, pleural disease, and lung mass with occupational, household, neighborhood, and slate roof-dense area residential asbestos exposure. International Journal of Environmental Research and Public Health. 2018;**15**:E1638. DOI: 10.3390/ijerph15081638

[56] Miserocchi G, Sancini G, MantegazzaF, ChiappinoG. Translocation pathways for inhaled asbestos fibers. Environmental Health. 2008;**7**:4. DOI: 10.1186/1476-069X-7-4

[57] Helmig S, Aliahmadi N, Schneider J. Tumour necrosis factor-alpha gene polymorphisms in asbestos-induced diseases. Biomarkers. 2010;**15**:400-409. DOI: 10.3109/1354750X.2010.481365

[58] Helmig S, Belwe A, Schneider J. Association of transforming growth factor beta1 gene polymorphisms and asbestos-induced fibrosis and tumors. Journal of Investigative Medicine. 2009;**57**:655-661. DOI: 10.2310/JIM.0b013e3181a4f32a

[59] Franko A, Dodic-Fikfak M, Arnerić N, Dolzan V. Glutathione S-transferases GSTM1 and GSTT1 polymorphisms and asbestosis. Journal of Occupational and Environmental Medicine. 2007;**49**:667-671

[60] Franko A, Dolžan V, Arnerić N, Dodič-Fikfak M. The influence of gene-gene and gene-environment interactions on the risk of asbestosis. BioMed Research International. 2013;**2013**:405743. DOI: 10.1155/2013/405743

[61] Raghu G, Weycker D, Edelsberg J, Bradford WZ, Oster G. Incidence and

prevalence of idiopathic pulmonary fibrosis. American Journal of Respiratory and Critical Care Medicine. 2006;**174**:810-816

[62] Kawabata Y, Shimizu Y, Hoshi A, et al. Asbestos exposure increases the incidence of usual interstitial pneumonia. Histopathology. 2016;**68**:339-346. DOI: 10.1111/his.12751

[63] Barber CM, Wiggans RE, Young C, Fishwick D. UK asbestos imports and mortality due to idiopathic pulmonary fibrosis. Occupational Medicine. 2016;**66**:106-111. DOI: 10.1093/occmed/kqv142

[64] Barber CM, Wiggans RE, Fishwick D. Estimating lifetime asbestos exposure in patients with idiopathic pulmonary fibrosis. The Annals of Occupational Hygiene. 2016;**60**: 649-650. DOI: 10.1093/annhyg/mew017

[65] Antao VC, Pinheiro GA, Wassell JT. Asbestosis mortality in the USA: Facts and predictions. Occupational and Environmental Medicine. 2009;**66**: 335-338. DOI: 10.1136/oem.2008.039172

[66] Kawabata Y, Watanabe T, Yamamura J, et al. A case of asbestosis without typical asbestos bodies. Nihon Kyōbu Shikkan Gakkai zasshi. 1985;**23**:1177-1183

[67] Iwai K, Mori T, Yamada N, Yamaguchi M, Hosoda Y. Idiopathic pulmonary fibrosis. Epidemiologic approaches to occupational exposure. American Journal of Respiratory and Critical Care Medicine. 1994;**150**:670-675

[68] Baumgartner KB, Samet JM, Coultas DB, et al. Occupational and environmental risk factors for idiopathic pulmonary fibrosis: A multicenter case-control study. Collaborating Centers. American Journal of Epidemiology. 2000;**152**:307-315

[69] Hubbard R, Cooper M, Antoniak M, et al. Risk of cryptogenic fibrosing alveolitis in metal workers. Lancet. 2000;**355**:466-467

[70] Pinheiro GA, Antao VC, Wood JM, Wassell JT. Occupational risks for idiopathic pulmonary fibrosis mortality in the United States. International Journal of Occupational and Environmental Health. 2008;**14**:117-123. DOI: 10.1179/oeh.2008.14.2.117

[71] Ley B, Collard HR. Epidemiology of idiopathic pulmonary fibrosis. Clinical Epidemiology. 2013;**5**:483-492. DOI: 10.2147/CLEP.S54815

[72] Ekström M, Gustafson T, Boman K, et al. Effects of smoking, gender and occupational exposure on the risk of severe pulmonary fibrosis: A population-based case-control study. British Medical Journal Open. 2014;**4**:e004018. DOI: 10.1136/bmjopen-2013-004018

[73] Gulati M, Redlich CA. Asbestosis and environmental causes of usual interstitial pneumonia. Current Opinion in Pulmonary Medicine. 2015;**21**:193-200. DOI: 10.1097/MCP.0000000000000144

[74] Armanios MY, Chen JJ, Cogan JD, et al. Telomerase mutations in families with idiopathic pulmonary fibrosis. The New England Journal of Medicine. 2007;**356**:1317-1326

[75] Alder JK, Chen JJ, Lancaster L, et al. Short telomeres are a risk factor for idiopathic pulmonary fibrosis. Proceedings of the National Academy of Sciences of the United States of America. 2008;**105**:13051-13056. DOI: 10.1073/pnas.0804280105

[76] Kropski JA, Pritchett JM, Zoz DF, et al. Extensive phenotyping of individuals at risk for familial interstitial pneumonia reveals clues to the pathogenesis of interstitial lung disease. American Journal of Respiratory and Critical Care Medicine.

2015;**191**:417-426. DOI: 10.1164/rccm.201406-1162OC

[77] Seibold MA, Wise AL, Speer MC, et al. A common MUC5B promoter polymorphism and pulmonary fibrosis. The New England Journal of Medicine. 2011;**364**:1503-1512

[78] Newton CA, Oldham JM, Ley B, et al. Telomere length and genetic variant associations with interstitial lung disease progression and survival. The European Respiratory Journal. 2019;**53**:1801641. DOI: 10.1183/13993003.01641-2018

[79] Arakawa H, Johkoh T, Honma K, et al. Chronic interstitial pneumonia in silicosis and mix-dust pneumoconiosis: Its prevalence and comparison of CT findings with idiopathic pulmonary fibrosis. Chest. 2007;**131**:1870-1876

[80] McConnochie K, Green FHY, Vallyathan V, et al. Interstitial fibrosis in coal workers: Experience in Wales and West Virginia. In: Dodgson J, McCallum RI, Bailey MR, et al., editors. British Occupational Hygiene Society 6th International Symposium. Cambridge, UK: Pergamon Press; 1988. pp. 553-560

[81] Honma K, Chiyotani K. Diffuse interstitial fibrosis in nonasbestos pneumoconiosis—A pathological study. Respiration. 1993;**60**:120-126

[82] Katabami M, Dosaka-Akita H, Honma K, et al. Pneumoconiosis-related lung cancers: Preferential occurrence from diffuse interstitial fibrosis-type pneumoconiosis. American Journal of Respiratory and Critical Care Medicine. 2000;**162**:295-300

[83] Arakawa H, Fujimoto K, Honma K, et al. Progression from near-normal to end-stage lungs in chronic interstitial pneumonia related to silica exposure: Long-term CT observations. AJR. American Journal of Roentgenology. 2008;**191**:1040-1045. DOI: 10.2214/AJR.07.3871

[84] Tanaka J, Moriyama H, Terada M, et al. An observational study of giant cell interstitial pneumonia and lung fibrosis in hard metal lung disease. BMJ Open. 2014;**4**:e004407. DOI: 10.1136/bmjopen-2013-004407

[85] Akashi T, Takemura T, Ando N, et al. Histopathologic analysis of sixteen autopsy cases of chronic hypersensitivity pneumonitis and comparison with idiopathic pulmonary fibrosis/usual interstitial pneumonia. American Journal of Clinical Pathology. 2009;**131**:405-415. DOI: 10.1309/AJCPNWX4SLZRP9SW

[86] Takemura T, Akashi T, Kamiya H, et al. Pathological differentiation of chronic hypersensitivity pneumonitis from idiopathic pulmonary fibrosis/usual interstitial pneumonia. Histopathology. 2012;**61**:1026-1035. DOI: 10.1111/j.1365-2559.2012.04322.x

[87] Churg A, Bilawich A, Wright JL. Pathology of chronic hypersensitivity pneumonitis what is it? What are the diagnostic criteria? Why do we care? Archives of Pathology & Laboratory Medicine. 2018;**142**:109-119. DOI: doi.org/10.5858/arpa.2017-0173-RA

[88] Ley B, Torgerson DG, Oldham JM, et al. Rare protein-altering telomere-related gene variants in patients with chronic hypersensitivity pneumonitis. American Journal of Respiratory and Critical Care Medicine. 3 July 2019. DOI: 10.1164/rccm.201902-0360OC

[89] Solomon JJ, Brown KK. Rheumatoid arthritis-associated interstitial lung disease. Open access Rheumatology: Research and Reviews. 2012;**4**:21-31

[90] Yunt ZX, Chung JH, Hobbs S, et al. High resolution computed tomography pattern of usual interstitial pneumonia in rheumatoid arthritis-associated interstitial lung disease: Relationship to survival. Respiratory Medicine. 2017;**126**:100-104. DOI: 10.1016/j.rmed.2017.03.027

[91] Spagnolo P, Lee JS, Sverzellati N, Rossi G, Cottin V. The lung in rheumatoid arthritis: Focus on interstitial lung disease. Arthritis & Rhematology. 2018;**70**:1544-1554. DOI: 10.1002/art.40574

[92] Singh N, Varghese J, England BR, et al. Impact of the pattern of interstitial lung disease on mortality in rheumatoid arthritis: A systematic literature review and meta-analysis. Seminars in Arthritis and Rheumatism. 15 May 2019. pii: S0049-0172(18)30639-5. DOI: 10.1016/j.semarthrit.2019.04.005

[93] Song JW, Do KH, Kim MY, Jang SJ, Colby TV, Kim DS. Pathologic and radiologic differences between idiopathic and collagen vascular disease-related usual interstitial pneumonia. Chest. 2009;**136**:23-30. DOI: 10.1378/chest.08-2572

[94] Juge PA, Lee JS, Ebstein E, et al. *MUC5B* promoter variant and rheumatoid arthritis with interstitial lung disease. The New England Journal of Medicine. 2018;**379**:2209-2219. DOI: 10.1056/NEJMoa1801562

Chapter 4

Immunocheckpoint Blockade in Malignant Pleural Mesothelioma

Nobukazu Fujimoto

Abstract

Targeting immunocheckpoint with immunomodulatory monoclonal antibodies has proven to be an effective antitumor strategy across a variety of cancers. The immunosuppressive tumor microenvironment in malignant pleural mesothelioma (MPM) has suggested that MPM might benefit from this kind of immunotherapy. In recent years, immunocheckpoint inhibitors (ICIs) have shown encouraging results for patients with MPM. Antibodies against programmed death 1 (PD-1) and PD-ligand 1 (PD-L1) have demonstrated favorable response, progression-free survival, and overall survival. The toxicity profiles were similar to those observed with ICIs in other malignancies, like melanoma and non-small cell lung cancer, and they appeared to be manageable. Nivolumab, an anti-PD-1 antibody, was approved in Japan for advanced or metastatic MPM patients resistant or intolerant to other chemotherapies. Important future issues include developing a combination therapy, where ICIs are combined with other agents (including other ICIs), and developing biomarkers for determining which patients might respond well and which might experience unacceptable toxicities.

Keywords: durvalumab, immunocheckpoint, nivolumab, pembrolizumab, PD-1

1. Introduction

Malignant pleural mesothelioma (MPM) is a rare pleural malignancy that is associated with asbestos exposure. Gemba et al. reported that more than 70% of malignant mesothelioma cases in Japan were associated with occupational or environmental asbestos exposure [1]. MPM is a highly aggressive neoplasm with a poor prognosis; the median overall survival (OS) is only about 12 months. Systemic chemotherapy with platinum plus pemetrexed is the recommended first-line systemic therapy for advanced MPM [2]. Some clinical trials have examined the efficacy of new agents to improve the results of the platinum/pemetrexed combination; however, no new agent has demonstrated significant clinical efficacy. Thus, the pemetrexed/platinum combination remains the standard treatment.

Currently, there is no recommended treatment option for MPM after first-line platinum/pemetrexed chemotherapy. Re-treatment with pemetrexed-based chemotherapy is a reasonable option for patients that achieved durable disease control with the first-line chemotherapy [3]. Other treatment options of salvage chemotherapy include vinorelbine and gemcitabine; however, the median OS with these agents only ranges from 5 to 10 months [4, 5]. Other experimental agents, such as angiogenesis inhibitors [6] or tyrosine kinase inhibitors [7], have not demonstrated efficacy.

Targeting immunocheckpoint with immunomodulatory monoclonal antibodies was shown to be an effective antitumor strategy across a variety of cancers [8]. The immunosuppressive tumor microenvironment in MPM has suggested that MPM might benefit from this kind of immunotherapy [9, 10]. In fact, in recent years, immunocheckpoint inhibitors (ICIs) have shown some encouraging results for patients with MPM.

In this chapter, we review recent clinical findings on several ICIs, including anti-cytotoxic T lymphocyte-associated antigen 4 (CTLA-4) antibody, anti-programmed death 1 (PD-1) antibody, and anti-PD-ligand 1 (PD-L1) antibody, for treating patients with MPM.

2. Anti-CTLA-4 antibody

Anti-CTLA-4 antibody was the first ICI described for treating MPM. Phase II studies demonstrated that tremelimumab, a selective human monoclonal antibody against CTLA-4, showed favorable activity as a second-line treatment for MPM [11, 12]. However, a double-blind study that compared tremelimumab to placebo in subjects with previously treated, unresectable malignant mesothelioma (DETERMINE study) failed to demonstrate differences in OS or progression-free survival (PFS) between the treatment and placebo groups [13]. After that, anti-CTLA-4 antibodies were studied in combination with an anti-PD-1 or anti-PD-L1 antibody.

3. Anti-PD-L1 antibody

Avelumab is a human IgG1 monoclonal antibody that targets PD-L1 [14]. A phase 1b open-label study (JAVELIN solid tumor) was conducted in patients with unresectable mesothelioma that progressed after platinum/pemetrexed treatment; patients were enrolled at 25 sites in three countries [15]. Of 53 patients treated, the objective response rate (RR) was 9% (95% confidence interval [95%CI]: 3.1–20.7%); one patient experienced a complete response, and four patients experienced a partial response. Responses were durable (median, 15.2 months; 95%CI: 11.1 to non-estimable) and occurred in patients with PD-L1-positive tumors (RR: 19%; 95%CI: 4.0–45.6) and PD-L1-negative tumors (RR: 7%; 95%CI: 0.9–24.3), based on a 5% or greater cutoff for PD-L1 expression. The median PFS was 4.1 months (95%CI: 1.4–6.2), and the 12-month PFS rate was 17.4% (95%CI: 7.7–30.4). The median OS was 10.7 months (95%CI: 6.4–20.2).

4. Anti-PD-1 antibody

4.1 Pembrolizumab

A nonrandomized, phase Ib trial was conducted to test pembrolizumab in patients with PD-1-positive MPM that had been treated previously. In the preliminary report, 20% of patients experienced an objective response, 72% experienced disease control, and the median OS was 18 months (95%CI: 9.4 to non-estimable) [16]. Then, a phase II trial assessed pembrolizumab activity in 65 unselected patients with MPM [17]. The objective RR was 19% and the disease control rate was 66%. The median PFS was 4.5 months (95%CI: 2.3–6.2), and the median OS was 11.5 months (95%CI: 7.6–14).

After those promising results, pembrolizumab was used off-label in Switzerland and Australia [18]. A total of 93 patients (48 from Switzerland and 45 from Australia) were treated. In those cohorts, the overall RR was 18%, the median PFS was 3.1 months, and the median OS was 7.2 months. Among patients with the non-epithelioid histological subtype, pembrolizumab treatment improved the objective RR (24% vs. 16%; $p = 0.54$) and the median PFS (5.6 vs. 2.8 months; $p = 0.02$).

4.2 Nivolumab

Another anti-PD-1 antibody, nivolumab, was first tested in recurrent MPM in the Netherlands [19]. In that single-center trial, patients with MPM received 3 mg/kg intravenous nivolumab every 2 weeks. Of the 34 patients included, eight patients (24%) displayed a partial response and another eight displayed stable disease, which resulted in a disease control rate of 47%. Japanese investigators also evaluated the efficacy and safety of nivolumab for advanced MPM in patients that were resistant or intolerant to prior chemotherapy [20]. Thirty-four patients were enrolled, and 10 patients (29.4%, 95%CI: 16.8–46.2) showed an objective response in a central assessment. Objective RRs were 25.9, 66.7, and 25.0% for epithelioid, sarcomatous, and biphasic histological subtypes, respectively (**Figure 1**). The median OS and PFS were 17.3 and 6.1 months, respectively (**Figure 2a** and **b**). Based on these findings,

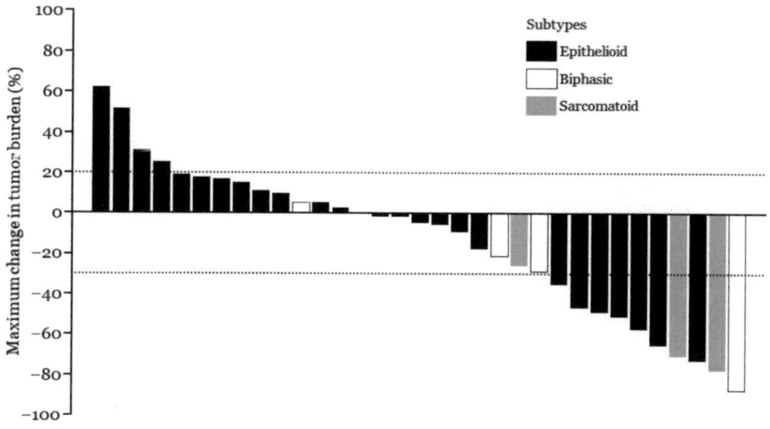

Figure 1.
A waterfall plot of the MERIT study results, which demonstrates the maximum percentage changes compared to baseline in target lesions of each patient, according to histological subtype (Ref. [20]).

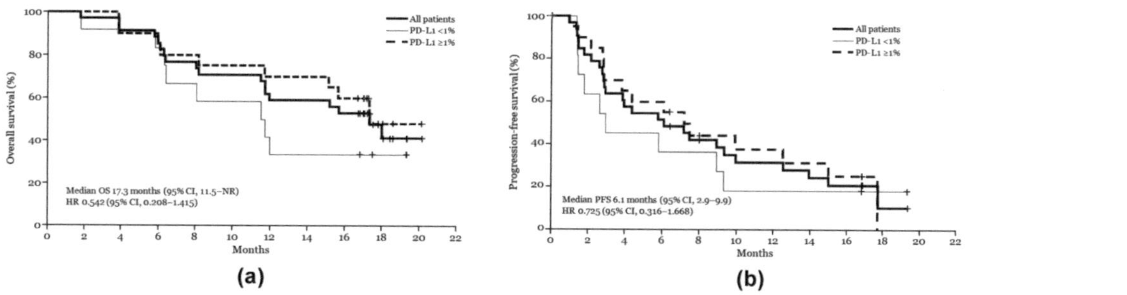

Figure 2.
Kaplan-Meier curves show survival for all patients and for patients grouped according to programmed death-ligand 1 (PD-L1) expression in the MERIT study (Ref. [20]). (a) Overall survival (OS); (b) progression-free survival (PFS). HRs compare the PD-L1 ≥ 1% group to the <1% group. CI, confidence interval; HR, hazard ratio; NR, not reached.

nivolumab was approved in Japan for patients with advanced or metastatic MPM that are resistant or intolerant to previous chemotherapy.

Although the effect requires confirmation in larger clinical trials, nivolumab and pembrolizumab might offer hope for patients with MPM.

5. Toxicity

The toxicity of these ICIs was acceptable in MPM. A study on pembrolizumab toxicity found grade 3 and 4 events, including adrenal insufficiency (3%), pneumonitis (3%), skin rash (3%), colitis (1.6%), confusion (1.6%), hepatitis (1.6%), and hyperglycemia (1.6%), and one grade 5 event of hepatitis (1.6%) [17]. In a study on nivolumab, adverse events of any grade occurred in 26 patients (76%), including fatigue (29%) and pruritus (15%) [19]. In that study, treatment-related grade 3 and 4 adverse events were reported in nine patients (26%); most events were pneumonitis, gastrointestinal disorders, and laboratory disorders. One treatment-related death was due to pneumonitis, but it was probably initiated by concurrent amiodarone therapy. These toxicity profiles were similar to those observed in other malignancies, including melanoma and non-small cell lung cancer (NSCLC), and they appeared to be manageable.

6. Future perspectives

Based on the promising results described above, ICIs could play a primary role in the treatment of MPM. An important issue for the future is whether ICIs can be combined with other agents, including other ICIs. For example, given the synergy between the PD-1/PD-L1 and CTLA-4 pathways in T-cell activation, a combination treatment with antibodies that target PD-1 or PD-L1 and CTLA-4 warrants investigation [22].

NIBIT-MESO-1 was an open-label, nonrandomized, phase II study that investigated the efficacy and safety of first- or second-line tremelimumab, a monoclonal antibody against CTLA-4, combined with durvalumab, a monoclonal antibody against PD-L1 [23]. In that study, patients with unresectable pleural or peritoneal mesothelioma received one dose of intravenous tremelimumab and durvalumab delivered every 4 weeks, for a total of four doses. This was followed by maintenance treatment with intravenous durvalumab. Of 40 patients, 11 (28%) displayed an objective response. The median PFS was 5.7 months (95%CI: 1.7–9.7), and the median OS was 16.6 months (95%CI: 13.1–20.1). Toxicity related to treatment was generally manageable and reversible.

Another multicenter, randomized, phase II study was conducted in France [24]. In that study, patients were randomly allocated to nivolumab or nivolumab plus ipilimumab. In the intention-to-treat population, the primary endpoint, 12-week disease control, was achieved by 25 (40%; 95%CI: 28–52) of 63 patients in the nivolumab group and by 32 (52%; 95%CI: 39–64) of 62 patients in the combination group. The most frequent grade 3 adverse events were asthenia (N = one [2%] with nivolumab vs. three [5%] with the combination), an asymptomatic increase in aspartate aminotransferase or alanine aminotransferase (N = none with nivolumab vs. four [7%] of each with the combination), and an asymptomatic increase in lipase (N = two [3%] with nivolumab vs. one [2%] with the combination). These findings indicated that the combination of anti-CTLA-4 and anti-PD1/PD-L1 antibodies appeared to be active and had a good safety profile in patients with MPM. Currently, there is an ongoing phase III, randomized, open-label trial for testing nivolumab in combination with ipilimumab vs. pemetrexed with cisplatin or carboplatin as a first-line therapy in unresectable MPM. The primary endpoint of the study, OS, will be reported in the near future.

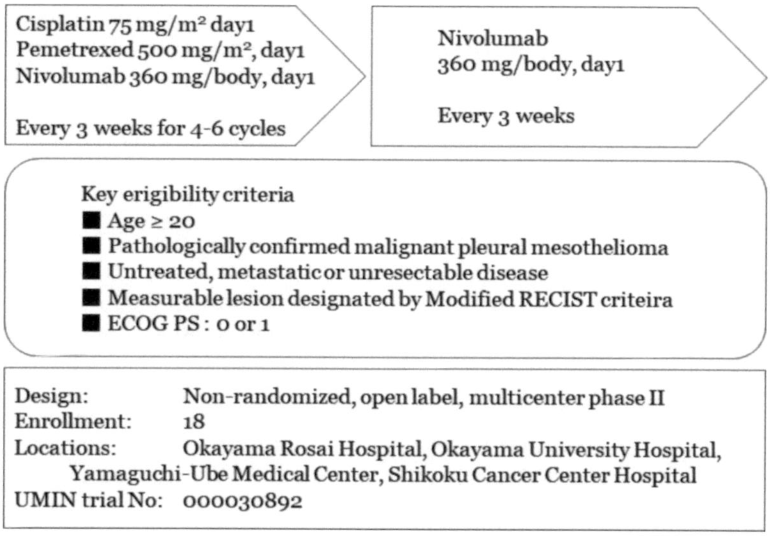

Figure 3.
Overview of a phase II trial for testing a first-line combination chemotherapy with cisplatin/pemetrexed and nivolumab for treating unresectable malignant pleural mesothelioma (Ref. [21]). RECIST, response evaluation criteria in solid tumors; ECOG, eastern cooperative oncology group; PS, performance status.

The combination of an anti-PD-1/PD-L1 antibody and conventional chemotherapy is also under investigation. Nowak et al. presented results from a phase II trial that tested durvalumab combined with cisplatin/pemetrexed in MPM [25]. The primary endpoint, PFS at 6 months, was 57% (N = 31/54; 95%CI: 45–68), the median PFS time was 6.9 months (95%CI: 5.5–9.0), and the objective RR was 48% (95%CI: 35–61). Grade 3–5 adverse events occurred in 36 patients, including neutropenia in 13%, nausea in 11%, anemia in 7%, fatigue in 6%, and any grade of peripheral neuropathy in 35%. The authors have conducted another phase II study to test the combination of nivolumab and cisplatin/pemetrexed, which is currently in progress (**Figure 3**) [21]. A large-scale randomized study for testing the combination of pembrolizumab and cisplatin/pemetrexed is also in progress. Based on whether these combination regimens, which include anti-PD1/PD-L1 antibodies, demonstrate sufficient activity, safety, and tolerability as first-line treatments, the standard regimen of cisplatin/pemetrexed might be replaced.

Another important issue is whether biomarkers can be developed to determine which patients might expect a response and which might expect unacceptable toxicity. Previous studies in patients with MPM have shown that tumors with positive PD-L1 expression were associated with worse survival outcomes compared to those with negative PD-L1 expression [26]. Although an optimal PD-L1 expression threshold could not be identified, a trend was observed, where a higher RR and more durable PFS were associated with increasing PD-L1 expression, in studies on pembrolizumab [17, 18] and nivolumab [20]. In some neoplasms, the tumor mutation burden or the tumor microenvironment was associated with the response to ICIs; however, those associations have not been established as biomarkers in MPM.

7. Conclusion

The prognosis of MPM remains poor. Recent encouraging results have suggested that a PD-1/PD-L1 blockade might be an effective treatment option for MPM. Although the effect requires confirmation in larger clinical trials, nivolumab and pembrolizumab might offer hope for patients with MPM. Further study is warranted to develop more effective treatment strategies, such as combining ICI with other ICIs or with conventional chemotherapy, and to establish biomarkers for distinguishing patients that might respond to treatment from those likely to develop unacceptable toxicities.

Acknowledgements

This study was supported by grants-in-aid from the Ministry of Health, Labor, and Welfare, Japan.

Conflict of interest

The author received consultancy fees from Boehringer Ingelheim, Ono, Bristol-Myers Squibb, Kyorin, and Kissei, and honoraria or research funding from Hisamitsu, Chugai, Ono, Taiho, Boehringer Ingelheim, Bristol-Myers Squibb, Novartis, GlaxoSmithKline, and MSD.

Author details

Nobukazu Fujimoto
Department of Medical Oncology, Okayama Rosai Hospital, Okayama, Japan

*Address all correspondence to: nobufujimot@gmail.com

References

[1] Gemba K, Fujimoto N, Kato K, Aoe K, Takeshima Y, Inai K, et al. National survey of malignant mesothelioma and asbestos exposure in Japan. Cancer Science. 2012;**103**:483-490. DOI: 10.1111/j.1349-7006.2011.02165.x

[2] Vogelzang NJ, Rusthoven JJ, Symanowski J, Denham C, Kaukel E, Ruffie P, et al. Phase III study of pemetrexed in combination with cisplatin versus cisplatin alone in patients with malignant pleural mesothelioma. Journal of Clinical Oncology. 2003;**21**:2636-2644. DOI: 10.1200/JCO.2003.11.136

[3] Bearz A, Talamini R, Rossoni G, Santo A, de Pangher V, Fasola G, et al. Re-challenge with pemetrexed in advanced mesothelioma: A multi-institutional experience. BMC Research Notes. 2012;**5**:482. DOI: 10.1186/1756-0500-5-482

[4] Bibby AC, Tsim S, Kanellakis N, Ball H, Talbot DC, Blyth KG, et al. Malignant pleural mesothelioma: An update on investigation, diagnosis and treatment. European Respiratory Review. 2016;**25**:472-486. DOI: 10.1183/16000617.0063-2016

[5] Buikhuisen WA, Hiddinga BI, Baas P, van Meerbeeck JP. Second line therapy in malignant pleural mesothelioma: A systematic review. Lung Cancer. 2015;**89**:223-231. DOI: 10.1016/j.lungcan.2015.06.018

[6] Buikhuisen WA, Burgers JA, Vincent AD, Korse CM, van Klaveren RJ, Schramel FM, et al. Thalidomide versus active supportive care for maintenance in patients with malignant mesothelioma after first-line chemotherapy (NVALT 5): An open-label, multicentre, randomised phase 3 study. The Lancet Oncology. 2013;**14**:543-551. DOI: 10.1016/S1470-2045(13)70125-6

[7] Mathy A, Baas P, Dalesio O, van Zandwijk N.Limited efficacy of imatinib mesylate in malignant mesothelioma: A phase II trial. Lung Cancer. 2005;**50**:83-86. DOI: 10.1016/j.lungcan.2005.04.010

[8] Wilson RAM, Evans TRJ, Fraser AR, Nibbs RJB. Immune checkpoint inhibitors: New strategies to checkmate cancer. Clinical and Experimental Immunology. 2018;**191**:133-148. DOI: 10.1111/cei.13081

[9] Bograd AJ, Suzuki K, Vertes E, Colovos C, Morales EA, Sadelain M, et al. Immune responses and immunotherapeutic interventions in malignant pleural mesothelioma. Cancer Immunology, Immunotherapy. 2011;**60**:1509-1527. DOI: 10.1007/s00262-011-1103-6

[10] Hegmans JP, Hemmes A, Hammad H, Boon L, Hoogsteden HC, Lambrecht BN. Mesothelioma environment comprises cytokines and T-regulatory cells that suppress immune responses. The European Respiratory Journal. 2006;**27**:1086-1095. DOI: 10.1183/09031936.06.00135305

[11] Calabro L, Morra A, Fonsatti E, Cutaia O, Amato G, Giannarelli D, et al. Tremelimumab for patients with chemotherapy-resistant advanced malignant mesothelioma: An open-label, single-arm, phase 2 trial. The Lancet Oncology. 2013;**14**:1104-1111. DOI: 10.1016/S1470-2045(13)70381-4

[12] Calabro L, Morra A, Fonsatti E, Cutaia O, Fazio C, Annesi D, et al. Efficacy and safety of an intensified schedule of tremelimumab for chemotherapy-resistant malignant mesothelioma: An open-label, single-arm, phase 2 study. The Lancet Respiratory Medicine. 2015;**3**:301-309. DOI: 10.1016/S2213-2600(15)00092-2

[13] Maio M, Scherpereel A, Calabro L, Aerts J, Cedres Perez S, Bearz A, et al. Tremelimumab as second-line or third-line treatment in relapsed malignant mesothelioma (DETERMINE): A multicentre, international, randomised, double-blind, placebo-controlled phase 2b trial. The Lancet Oncology. 2017;**18**:1261-1273. DOI: 10.1016/S1470-2045(17)30446-1

[14] Heery CR, O'Sullivan-Coyne G, Madan RA, Cordes L, Rajan A, Rauckhorst M, et al. Avelumab for metastatic or locally advanced previously treated solid tumours (JAVELIN solid tumor): A phase 1a, multicohort, dose-escalation trial. The Lancet Oncology. 2017;**18**:587-598. DOI: 10.1016/S1470-2045(17)30239-5

[15] Hassan R, Thomas A, Nemunaitis JJ, Patel MR, Bennouna J, Chen FL, et al. Efficacy and safety of avelumab treatment in patients with advanced unresectable mesothelioma: Phase 1b results from the JAVELIN solid tumor trial. JAMA Oncology. 2019;**5**:351-357. DOI: 10.1001/jamaoncol.2018.5428

[16] Alley EW, Lopez J, Santoro A, Morosky A, Saraf S, Piperdi B, et al. Clinical safety and activity of pembrolizumab in patients with malignant pleural mesothelioma (KEYNOTE-028): Preliminary results from a non-randomised, open-label, phase 1b trial. The Lancet Oncology. 2017;**18**:623-630. DOI: 10.1016/S1470-2045(17)30169-9

[17] Desai A, Karrison T, Rose B, Tan Y, Hill B, Pemberton E, et al. Phase II trial of pembrolizumab (NCT02399371) in previously-treated malignant mesothelioma: Final analysis. Journal of Thoracic Oncology. 2018;**13**:S339

[18] Metaxas Y, Rivalland G, Mauti LA, Klingbiel D, Kao S, Schmid S, et al. Pembrolizumab as palliative immunotherapy in malignant pleural mesothelioma. Journal of Thoracic Oncology. 2018;**13**:1784-1791. DOI: 10.1016/j.jtho.2018.08.007

[19] Quispel-Janssen J, van der Noort V, de Vries JF, Zimmerman M, Lalezari F, Thunnissen E, et al. Programmed death 1 blockade with nivolumab in patients with recurrent malignant pleural mesothelioma. Journal of Thoracic Oncology. 2018;**13**:1569-1576

[20] Okada M, Kijima T, Aoe K, Kato T, Fujimoto N, Nakagawa K, et al. Clinical efficacy and safety of nivolumab: Results of a multicenter, open-label, single-arm, Japanese phase 2 study in malignant pleural mesothelioma (MERIT). Clinical Cancer Research. 2019. DOI: 10.1158/1078-0432.CCR-19-0103. pii: clincanres.0103.2019

[21] Fujimoto N, Aoe K, Kozuki T, Oze I, Kato K, Kishimoto T, et al. A phase II trial of first-line combination chemotherapy with cisplatin, pemetrexed, and nivolumab for unresectable malignant pleural mesothelioma: A study protocol. Clinical Lung Cancer. 2018;**19**:e705-e707. DOI: 10.1016/j.cllc.2018.05.001

[22] Das R, Verma R, Sznol M, Boddupalli CS, Gettinger SN, Kluger H, et al. Combination therapy with anti-CTLA-4 and anti-PD-1 leads to distinct immunologic changes in vivo. Journal of Immunology. 2015;**194**:950-959. DOI: 10.4049/jimmunol.1401686

[23] Calabro L, Morra A, Giannarelli D, Amato G, D'Incecco A, Covre A, et al. Tremelimumab combined with durvalumab in patients with mesothelioma (NIBIT-MESO-1): An open-label, non-randomised, phase 2 study. The Lancet Respiratory Medicine. 2018;**6**:451-460. DOI: 10.1016/S2213-2600(18)30151-6

[24] Scherpereel A, Mazieres J, Greillier L, Lantuejoul S, Do P, Bylicki O, et al. French Cooperative Thoracic, Intergroup. Nivolumab or

nivolumab plus ipilimumab in patients with relapsed malignant pleural mesothelioma (IFCT-1501 MAPS2): A multicentre, open-label, randomised, non-comparative, phase 2 trial. The Lancet Oncology. 2019;**20**:239-253. DOI: 10.1016/S1470-2045(18)30765-4

[25] Nowak AKP, Lesterhuis W, Hughes B, Brown C, Kao S, Karikios D, et al. DREAM—A phase 2 trial of durvalumab with first line chemotherapy in mesothelioma: Final result. Journal of Thoracic Oncology. 2018;**13**(10, Supplement):S338-S3S9

[26] Cedres S, Ponce-Aix S, Zugazagoitia J, Sansano I, Enguita A, Navarro-Mendivil A, et al. Analysis of expression of programmed cell death 1 ligand 1 (PD-L1) in malignant pleural mesothelioma (MPM). PLoS One. 2015;**10**:e0121071. DOI: 10.1371/journal.pone.0121071

Chapter 5

Potential Roles of Matrix Metalloproteinases in Malignant Mesothelioma

Shibo Ying, Yanbin Wang and Lyuyang Lyu

Abstract

Malignant mesothelioma (MM) is a rare, aggressive, and highly lethal cancer that is primary induced by exposure to asbestos fibers. Matrix metalloproteinases (MMPs) are a family of zinc-dependent endopeptidases that are involved in metastasis, and their overexpression correlates with tumor cell invasion and metastasis because they degrade the extracellular matrix (ECM) and process adhesion and cytoskeletal proteins, growth factors, chemokines, and cytokines. Recent evidence has shown that MMPs participate in MM progression, indicating that they are potential novel biomarkers and attractive targets for cancer therapy. In this chapter, we will describe MMPs in carcinogenic mechanisms based on in vivo and in vitro experimental evidence, outline the clinical findings, and speculate the possible roles of MMPs in MM.

Keywords: malignant mesothelioma, matrix metalloproteinases, mesothelial carcinogenesis, extracellular matrix, biomarker

1. Introduction

Malignant mesothelioma (MM) is a rare, aggressive cancer that originates from mesothelial tissue in the pleura, peritoneum, and pericardium; MM has been associated with asbestos exposure, especially in occupational settings [1]. In some countries, such as Turkey and Japan, MM is also due to environmental asbestos exposure, which affects people who live in the vicinity of natural asbestos mines or factories that use asbestos [2–4]. Mesothelioma is highly resistant to conventional cancer therapies. MM patients usually have a poor prognosis, with a median survival of 12–18 months, due to the lack of effective treatments and difficulty in diagnosing this disease at the early stage [5–7]. In general, there are three main histological subtypes of mesothelioma. The epithelioid and sarcomatoid subtypes are characterized by cuboid and fibroblastoid cells, respectively. The biphasic subtype contains a mixture of both cell types and confers the worst prognosis. The most widely used treatments for MM are surgery with or without adjuvant chemotherapy and/or radiotherapy [8]. The first-line treatment option for unresectable MM is chemotherapy with cisplatin plus pemetrexed [9, 10]. Nevertheless, MM may be resistant to these conventional therapeutic approaches, and palliative care strategies are controversial. Although crocidolite and/or chrysotile have not been used for more than 10 years in many developed and developing countries, high mortality rates associated with mesothelioma persist since the clinical manifestations of MM are insidious and nonspecific. It is worth noting that MM has a long latency period (mean, 30–40 years) from the time of asbestos exposure to tumorigenesis [4, 11]. Thus, valuable biomarkers for the prediction or diagnosis of MM at early stages, prognostic markers, and novel therapeutic strategies are urgently needed.

Matrix metalloproteinases (MMPs, also known as matrixins) are a family of zinc-dependent endopeptidases that degrade all components of the extracellular matrix (ECM); thus, MMPs are involved in ECM remodeling. In addition to functioning as the main ECM regulators, MMPs also modulate intra- and extracellular signaling pathways and networks through the proteolytic processing of various biomolecules. The first MMP was reported by Gross and Lapiere as a collagenase engaged in tail resorption during tadpole metamorphosis [12]. To date, 24 MMP genes, including a gene duplication, that encode 23 unique MMP proteins have been identified in humans [13, 14]. According to substrate specificity, sequence similarity, and specific role, MMPs can be divided into eight main groups: (1) collagenases (MMP-1, MMP-8, and MMP-13), (2) matrilysins (MMP-7 and MMP-26), (3) metalloelastase (MMP-12), (4) stromelysins (MMP-3, MMP-10, and MMP-11), (5) gelatinases (MMP-2 and MMP-9); (6) enamelysin (MMP-20); (7) membrane-type MMPs (MMP-14, MMP-15, MMP-16, MMP-17, MMP-24, and MMP-25), and (8) others (MMP-19, MMP-21, MMP-23, MMP-27, and MMP-28) [13, 15]. Interestingly, the proteolytic activities of MMPs are precisely controlled by activation of their precursors and inhibition by endogenous inhibitors, α-macroglobulins, and tissue inhibitors of metalloproteinases [13]. Except for six membrane-associated MMPs, the other 17 MMPs are soluble secreted enzymes [16]. In addition, growth factors, chemokines, and cytokines modulate the expression of MMPs through various pathways to affect ECM degradation and, in turn, influence growth factors, which ultimately affect cancer cell migration and invasion [17, 18].

Of note, MMPs are expressed in various cancer tissues, and their expression levels are closely associated with the properties of invasive growth and metastasis [15]. Accumulating evidence suggests that ECM degradation by MMPs at the cell surface enhances tumor growth, invasion, and metastasis through the proteolytic degradation of ECM, altered cell-cell, and cell-ECM interactions and effects on cell migration and angiogenesis [17, 19]. More recently, the roles of different MMPs have become increasingly studied in the field of MM research. Experimental evidence indicates that MMP-1, MMP-2, and MMP-9 are involved in mesothelial carcinogenesis. Several MMPs, such as MMP-7, MMP-14, and MMP-9, are potential biomarkers for MM. In the following sections, we will describe the roles of MMPs in carcinogenic mechanisms based on in vivo and in vitro experimental evidence, outline the clinical findings, and highlight the possible roles of MMPs in MM, as well as future prospects.

2. Crucial roles of MMPs in mesothelial carcinogenesis

Some MMPs are upregulated and considered mesenchymal markers of epithelial-to-mesenchymal transition (EMT), such as MMP-1, MMP-2, and MMP-9 [20]. EMT not only is associated with many physiological processes, such as embryonic development, but also plays a vital role in pathological processes, including cancer cell invasion and migration [21–23]. During EMT, epithelial cells lose their phenotype and acquire a mesenchymal phenotype, including the loss of cell polarity and cell adhesion in cell-cell and cell-basement membrane interactions and the acquisition of ECM degradation ability, which is directly related to MMPs. Currently, published studies implicate MMPs as inducers of EMT during MM progression. In addition, MMPs play a mediator role in cellular signaling pathways controlled by growth factors and cytokines [17, 24]. Here, we describe these two main roles of MMPs in MM carcinogenesis. Moreover, we propose possible mechanisms involving MMPs, as shown in **Figure 1**.

2.1 EMT inducer

MMP-1 is an interstitial collagenase that specifically targets the degradation of collagen types I–III [25]. Schelch et al. reported that in malignant pleural mesothelioma (MPM) cells in vitro, fibroblast growth factor 2(FGF2) and epidermal growth factor (EGF) may induce EMT via mitogen-activated protein kinase kinase (MEK)/ MMP-1 signaling [26]. The experimental results indicated that MMP-1 inhibition by the pan-MMP inhibitor GM6001 or transfection with siRNAs targeting MMP-1 could prevent FGF2-induced cell scattering and invasion in the M38K cell line (a biphasic MPM cell line) [26]. In MPM tissue specimens, higher MMP-1 expression was observed in the sarcomatoid compartment than in the epithelioid compartment. Normal pleura were weakly positive for MMP-1 [26]. These results suggest that MMP-1 causally contributes to sarcomatoid morphology and increases cell invasiveness during EMT.

MMP-2, also named gelatinase A, is expressed by almost all cell types, and its classical substrates are denatured collagen (gelatin) and basement membrane [25, 27]. Indeed, MMP-2 acts as a cancer-associated EMT inducer or modulator in a number of tumors, such as breast cancer [16, 28], hepatocellular carcinoma [29], prostate cancer [30], ovarian cancer [31], oral squamous cell carcinoma [32], and MM [33]. Regarding MM, MMP-2 secretion from human normal mesothelial MeT-5A cells increased upon treatment with chrysotile or transforming growth factor-β (TGF-β) [33], and EMT was induced. This in vitro experimental result of increased MMP-2 secretion by cells exposed to chrysotile asbestos suggests changes in the surrounding microenvironment that render the ECM more amenable to degradation and invasion [33, 34]. Of course, the underlying mechanism of MMP-2-induced EMT in MM development requires further study.

MMP-9 is a type IV collagenase also known as gelatinase B [35] that has a similar ability to cleave gelatin as MMP-2. MMP-9 has been recognized as an EMT mediator in cancer progression and appears to be a potential therapeutic target [35–37].

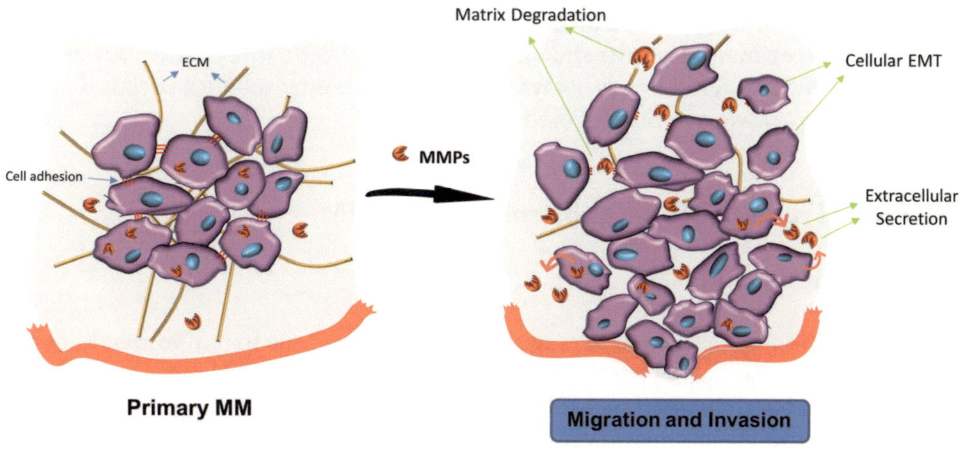

Figure 1.
Schematic representation of MMP-involved mechanisms in MM carcinogenesis. See detail in text. MM, malignant mesothelioma; EMT, epithelial-to-mesenchymal transition; ECM, extracellular matrix.

Elevated MMP-9 levels were observed in a 3D microtumor model of patient-derived mesothelioma cells, consistent with the elevated MMP-9 levels in patient breast tumors compared to healthy mammary glands [38]. Moreover, MMP-9 secreted into conditioned media by large microtumors induced a migratory phenotype in nonmigratory small microtumors, and blocking MMP-9 with GM6001 effectively abolished the collective migration of mesothelioma microtumors [38]. These findings imply that a self-regulated positive feedback loop involving MMP-9 is established during tumor progression and migration [38]. Additionally, the invasion of H2052 (mesothelioma cell line) and JP5 cells (primary mesothelioma cell line) into a 3D collagen matrix induced by gremlin-1 (a protein antagonist of bone morphogenetic proteins) was significantly alleviated by GM6001 and BB2516 (broad-spectrum MMP inhibitors) [39]. Interestingly, in our previous study, we found that serum MMP-2 and MMP-9 levels were correlated with each other in both healthy control and MM groups in a Han cohort from Eastern China [40]. Nevertheless, there were no significant differences in MMP-2/MMP-9 levels between the healthy control and MM groups.

2.2 Signaling pathway mediator

Various growth factors, cytokines, and miRNAs engage specific cellular signaling pathways, such as the MEK and extracellular signal-regulated kinase (ERK) signaling pathways, to regulate MMP expression levels to degrade the ECM, and MMPs then contribute to the release of tumor-related factors, such as vascular endothelial growth factor and TGF-β, from the ECM [17, 24].

MMP-1 expression showed an increasing trend in MM cell lines from no treatment to treatment with FGF2 and EGF and a pronounced decrease upon treatment with selumetinib (MEK inhibitor), suggesting that the growth factors FGF2 and EGF regulate MMP-1 expression via the MEK signaling pathway in MM [26]. TGF-β, another important growth factor that regulates cell growth and differentiation, affects MMP-2 expression in MeT-5A [33] and JL-1 cells [39]. Moreover, growth hormone-releasing hormone (GHRH) antagonists (MIA-602 and MIA-690) equally blunted MMP-2 and MMP-9 mRNA levels in both REN and MSTO-211H cells (MM cell lines), indirectly indicating that MMP-2/MMP-9 expression is induced by GHRH [41], as well as by adenosine diphosphate in ZL55 cells (an epithelioid MM cell line), via the nuclear factor kappa-B, protein kinase B, and ERK1/2 signaling pathways [42]. Interestingly, microtumor treated with GM6001 showed reduced pERK/ERK ratios and ERK activation [38]. Notably, miR-591 targets MMP-2 expression, and overexpression of miR-591 inhibited MMP-2 levels in MPM cells [43]. These experimental results show that MMP expression is regulated by various factors via multiple signaling pathways and that MMPs interact with such inducers and signaling pathways in MM carcinogenesis.

3. Potential roles of MMPs as biomarkers for MM

3.1 Pathological markers

To date, MM is still difficult to diagnose in early stages due to our limited knowledge of its molecular pathogenesis. Indeed, pathological examination techniques to diagnose MM and distinguish MM from other diseases must be improved [44]. However, more molecular markers are required to distinguish benign from malignant mesothelial disease or other tumors. In addition, effective pathologic predictors of prognosis and therapeutic response are urgently needed. Since MMPs are involved in tumor pathogenesis, some MMPs may be potential pathological markers.

In general, MMP expression and activation are very low and tightly regulated during normal tissue homeostasis. MMP production and activation are rapidly induced during active tissue remodeling and in pathological conditions such as cancer [37]. MMP-7 and MMP-14 are potential diagnostic and prognostic biomarkers of mesothelioma, respectively. MMP-7 is a highly specific negative biomarker to distinguish MM from other high-grade serous carcinomas with 100% specificity and moderate sensitivity, but it cannot distinguish mesothelial cells from reactive mesothelial cells in serous effusion due to uniformly negative expression of MMP-7 in reactive mesothelial cells [45]. It is intriguing that MMP-14 is a potential biomarker for the differential diagnosis of MPM and reactive mesothelial hyperplasia (MH). A group from Italy found that MMP-14 expression is markedly increased in MPM patient specimens compared with MH specimens based on polymerase chain reaction array and immunohistochemistry analyses [46]. MMP-14 levels have been reported to be elevated in all tissue samples from MM patients compared to those from normal individuals, but more evidence is needed to substantiate MMP-14 as a diagnostic biomarker for MM [47]. MMP-14 expression has prognostic value for MM. Clinically high MMP-14 expression in MM patients is significantly correlated with poor prognosis [47].

3.2 Genetic biomarkers

Although most mesotheliomas are attributable to asbestos exposure, genetic factors are also important causes of carcinogenesis. Gene mutations influence the prognosis of MM. For example, heritable mutations in BRCA1-associated protein-1 (BAP1), a tumor suppressor gene, may predispose individuals to asbestos-related MM [48, 49]. Moreover, Baumann et al. reported that mesothelioma patients with germline BAP1 mutations have a seven-fold improvement in long-term survival [50].

More recently, some MMP single-nucleotide polymorphisms (SNPs) have been found to have potential as genetic biomarkers for MM. For instance, Štrbac et al. reported that patients carrying a polymorphic MMP-9 rs2250889 allele had a negative outcome, with a shorter time to progression (TTP) (6.07 vs. 10.03 months, HR = 2.45, 95% CI = 1.45–4.14, p = 0.001) and worse overall survival (OS) (9.23 vs. 19.2 months, HR = 2.39, 95% CI = 1.37–4.18, p = 0.002) than those with the reference allele [51]. However, patients harboring at least one polymorphic MMP-9 rs20544 allele had a positive outcome, with a longer TTP (10.93 vs. 9.40 months, HR = 0.57, 95% CI = 0.38–0.86, p = 0.007) and improved OS (20.67 vs. 13.50 months, HR = 0.56, 95% CI = 0.37–0.85, p = 0.007) [51]. These researchers also found that the MMP-2 rs243865 polymorphism plays a protective role in MM; carriers of this polymorphism have a decreased risk for MM (OR = 0.66, 95% CI = 0.44–1.00, p = 0.050) [52]. Interestingly, the decreased risk for MM is more pronounced in people exposed to asbestos [52]. These findings provide insight into some MMP SNPs that are considered genetic biomarkers, indicate the prognosis of MM patients, and predict susceptibility to MM. In the future, appropriate genetic counseling and clinical management should be considered for MM patients who are carriers of MMP-2/MMP-9 susceptibility SNPs.

4. Conclusion

In this chapter, we provide an overview of recent findings on MMP function in MM and the mechanisms by which MMPs may induce both phenotypic and genotypic alterations that facilitate MM progression and invasion. Accumulating evidence indicates that tumor-associated MMPs can stimulate processes associated with EMT, a developmental event that is activated in MM cells during invasion and metastasis. Meanwhile, future investigations on extracellular targets and intracellular signaling pathways through which MMPs can induce EMT of MM cells will provide insight into novel therapeutic targets. We also describe possible roles of MMPs as pathological markers or genetic biomarkers in MM. Certainly, the underlying mechanisms of secreted MMPs, including their function and circulation, are complex in MM and remain to be elucidated in the future.

Acknowledgements

This study was supported by the National Natural Science Foundation of China (81502794, 81973011), the Qianjiang Talents Project of Zhejiang Province (QJD1602027), the Science and Technology Department of Zhejiang Province (1925D), the Zhejiang Provincial Natural Science Foundation of China (LY16H240001), the Health Commission of Zhejiang Province (2017PY015, 2018KY038), and the Science and Technology Project of Cixi City (CN2018023). The research assistance of Dr. Xing Zhang and Dr. Jianlin Lou is gratefully acknowledged.

Conflict of interest

The authors declare no conflicts of interest.

Author details

Shibo Ying*, Yanbin Wang and Lyuyang Lyu
Institute of Occupational Diseases, Zhejiang Academy of Medical Sciences, Hangzhou, China

*Address all correspondence to: shiboying@zjams.cn

References

[1] Takahashi K, Landrigan PJ, Collegium R. The global health dimensions of asbestos and asbestos-related diseases. Annals of Global Health. 2016;**82**(1):209-213. DOI: 10.1016/j.aogh.2016.01.019

[2] Metintas S, Batirel HF, Bayram H, Yilmaz U, Karadag M, Ak G, et al. Turkey national mesothelioma surveillance and environmental asbestos exposure control program. International Journal of Environmental Research and Public Health. 2017;**14**(11). DOI: 10.3390/ijerph14111293

[3] Berk S, Yalcin H, Dogan OT, Epozturk K, Akkurt I, Seyfikli Z. The assessmentofthemalignantmesothelioma cases and environmental asbestos exposure in Sivas province, Turkey. Environmental Geochemistry and Health. 2014;**36**(1):55-64. DOI: 10.1007/s10653-013-9518-y

[4] Zha L, Kitamura Y, Kitamura T, Liu R, Shima M, Kurumatani N, et al. Population-based cohort study on health effects of asbestos exposure in Japan. Cancer Science. 2019;**110**(3):1076-1084. DOI: 10.1111/cas.13930

[5] Bononi A, Napolitano A, Pass HI, Yang H, Carbone M. Latest developments in our understanding of the pathogenesis of mesothelioma and the design of targeted therapies. Expert Review of Respiratory Medicine. 2015;**9**(5):633-654. DOI: 10.1586/17476348.2015.1081066

[6] Bibby AC, Maskell NA. Current treatments and trials in malignant pleural mesothelioma. The Clinical Respiratory Journal. 2018;**12**(7):2161-2169. DOI: 10.1111/crj.12938

[7] Mutti L, Peikert T, Robinson BWS, Scherpereel A, Tsao AS, de Perrot M, et al. Scientific advances and new frontiers in mesothelioma therapeutics. Journal of Thoracic Oncology. 2018;**13**(9):1269-1283. DOI: 10.1016/j.jtho.2018.06.011

[8] Opitz I. Management of malignant pleural mesothelioma—The European experience. Journal of Thoracic Disease. 2014;**6**(Suppl 2):S238-S252. DOI: 10.3978/j.issn.2072-1439.2014.05.03

[9] Fujimoto N, Aoe K, Kozuki T, Oze I, Kato K, Kishimoto T, et al. A phase II trial of first-line combination chemotherapy with cisplatin, pemetrexed, and nivolumab for unresectable malignant pleural mesothelioma: A study protocol. Clinical Lung Cancer. 2018;**19**(5):e705-e707. DOI: 10.1016/j.cllc.2018.05.001

[10] Bibby AC, Tsim S, Kanellakis N, Ball H, Talbot DC, Blyth KG, et al. Malignant pleural mesothelioma: An update on investigation, diagnosis and treatment. European Respiratory Review. 2016;**25**(142):472-486. DOI: 10.1183/16000617.0063-2016

[11] Musk ABW, de Klerk N, Brims FJ. Mesothelioma in Australia: A review. Medical Journal of Australia. 2017;**207**(10):449-452

[12] Gross J, Lapiere CM. Collagenolytic activity in amphibian tissues: A tissue culture assay. Proceedings of the National Academy of Sciences of the United States of America. 1962;**48**:1014-1022. DOI: 10.1073/pnas.48.6.1014

[13] Khokha R, Murthy A, Weiss A. Metalloproteinases and their natural inhibitors in inflammation and immunity. Nature Reviews Immunology. 2013;**13**(9):649-665. DOI: 10.1038/nri3499

[14] Sabir N, Hussain T, Mangi MH, Zhao D, Zhou X. Matrix metalloproteinases: Expression,

regulation and role in the immunopathology of tuberculosis. Cell Proliferation. 2019;**2019**:e12649. DOI: 10.1111/cpr.12649

[15] Gobin E, Bagwell K, Wagner J, Mysona D, Sandirasegarane S, Smith N, et al. A pan-cancer perspective of matrix metalloproteases (MMP) gene expression profile and their diagnostic/prognostic potential. BMC Cancer. 2019;**19**(1):581. DOI: 10.1186/s12885-019-5768-0

[16] Radisky ES, Radisky DC. Matrix metalloproteinase-induced epithelial-mesenchymal transition in breast cancer. Journal of Mammary Gland Biology and Neoplasia. 2010;**15**(2):201-212. DOI: 10.1007/s10911-010-9177-x

[17] Tang H, Tang Z, Jiang Y, Wei W, Lu J. Pathological and therapeutic aspects of matrix metalloproteinases: Implications in osteosarcoma. Asia-Pacific Journal of Clinical Oncology. 2019;**15**(4):218-224. DOI: 10.1111/ajco.13165

[18] Chen Y, Peng S, Cen H, Lin Y, Huang C, Chen Y, et al. MicroRNA hsa-miR-623 directly suppresses MMP1 and attenuates IL-8-induced metastasis in pancreatic cancer. International Journal of Oncology. 2019;**55**(1):142-156. DOI: 10.3892/ijo.2019.4803

[19] Gialeli C, Theocharis AD, Karamanos NK. Roles of matrix metalloproteinases in cancer progression and their pharmacological targeting. The FEBS Journal. 2011;**278**(1):16-27. DOI: 10.1111/j.1742-4658.2010.07919.x

[20] Lamouille S, Xu J, Derynck R. Molecular mechanisms of epithelial-mesenchymal transition. Nature Reviews Molecular Cell Biology. 2014;**15**(3):178-196. DOI: 10.1038/nrm3758

[21] Thiery JP, Acloque H, Huang RY, Nieto MA. Epithelial-mesenchymal transitions in development and disease. Cell. 2009;**139**(5):871-890. DOI: 10.1016/j.cell.2009.11.007

[22] Singh S, Chakrabarti R. Consequences of EMT-driven changes in the immune microenvironment of breast cancer and therapeutic response of cancer cells. Journal of Clinical Medicine. 2019;**8**(5). DOI: 10.3390/jcm8050642

[23] Bonnomet A, Brysse A, Tachsidis A, Waltham M, Thompson EW, Polette M, et al. Epithelial-to-mesenchymal transitions and circulating tumor cells. Journal of Mammary Gland Biology and Neoplasia. 2010;**15**(2):261-273. DOI: 10.1007/s10911-010-9174-0

[24] Chang C, Werb Z. The many faces of metalloproteases: Cell growth, invasion, angiogenesis and metastasis. Trends in Cell Biology. 2001;**11**(11):S37-S43

[25] Craig VJ, Zhang L, Hagood JS, Owen CA. Matrix metalloproteinases as therapeutic targets for idiopathic pulmonary fibrosis. American Journal of Respiratory Cell and Molecular Biology. 2015;**53**(5):585-600. DOI: 10.1165/rcmb.2015-0020TR

[26] Schelch K, Wagner C, Hager S, Pirker C, Siess K, Lang E, et al. FGF2 and EGF induce epithelial-mesenchymal transition in malignant pleural mesothelioma cells via a MAPKinase/MMP1 signal. Carcinogenesis. 2018;**39**(4):534-545. DOI: 10.1093/carcin/bgy018

[27] Jobin PG, Butler GS, Overall CM. New intracellular activities of matrix metalloproteinases shine in the moonlight. Biochimica et Biophysica Acta-Molecular Cell Research. 2017;**1864**(11 Pt A):2043-2055. DOI: 10.1016/j.bbamcr.2017.05.013

[28] Qin H, Liu X, Li F, Miao L, Li T, Xu B, et al. PAD1 promotes epithelial-mesenchymal transition and metastasis

in triple-negative breast cancer cells by regulating MEK1-ERK1/2-MMP2 signaling. Cancer Letters. 2017;**409**:30-41. DOI: 10.1016/j.canlet.2017.08.019

[29] Ren T, Zhu L, Cheng M. CXCL10 accelerates EMT and metastasis by MMP-2 in hepatocellular carcinoma. American Journal of Translational Research. 2017;**9**(6):2824-2837

[30] Hafeez BB, Ganju A, Sikander M, Kashyap VK, Hafeez ZB, Chauhan N, et al. Ormeloxifene suppresses prostate tumor growth and metastatic phenotypes via inhibition of oncogenic beta-catenin signaling and EMT progression. Molecular Cancer Therapeutics. 2017;**16**(10):2267-2280. DOI: 10.1158/1535-7163.MCT-17-0157

[31] Chen Y, Huang L, Wang S, Li JL, Li M, Wu Y, et al. WFDC2 contributes to epithelial-mesenchymal transition (EMT) by activating AKT signaling pathway and regulating MMP-2 expression. Cancer Management and Research. 2019;**11**:2415-2424. DOI: 10.2147/CMAR.S192950

[32] Lee AY, Fan CC, Chen YA, Cheng CW, Sung YJ, Hsu CP, et al. Curcumin inhibits invasiveness and epithelial-mesenchymal transition in oral squamous cell carcinoma through reducing matrix metalloproteinase 2,9 and modulating p53-E-cadherin pathway. Integrative Cancer Therapies. 2015;**14**(5):484-490. DOI: 10.1177/1534735415588930

[33] Turini S, Bergandi L, Gazzano E, Prato M, Aldieri E. Epithelial to mesenchymal transition in human mesothelial cells exposed to asbestos fibers: Role of TGF-beta as mediator of malignant mesothelioma development or metastasis via EMT event. International Journal of Molecular Sciences. 2019;**20**(1). DOI: 10.3390/ijms20010150

[34] Simeone P, Trerotola M, Franck J, Cardon T, Marchisio M, Fournier I, et al. The multiverse nature of epithelial to mesenchymal transition. Seminars in Cancer Biology. 2018;**S1044-579X**(18): 30086-30095. DOI: 10.1016/j.semcancer.2018.11.004

[35] Vafadari B, Salamian A, Kaczmarek L. MMP-9 in translation: From molecule to brain physiology, pathology, and therapy. Journal of Neurochemistry. 2016;**139**(Suppl 2): 91-114. DOI: 10.1111/jnc.13415

[36] Knapinska AM, Estrada CA, Fields GB. The roles of matrix metalloproteinases in pancreatic cancer. Progress in Molecular Biology and Translational Science. 2017;**148**:339-354. DOI: 10.1016/bs.pmbts.2017.03.004

[37] Orlichenko LS, Radisky DC. Matrix metalloproteinases stimulate epithelial-mesenchymal transition during tumor development. Clinical & Experimental Metastasis. 2008;**25**(6):593-600. DOI: 10.1007/s10585-008-9143-9

[38] Singh M, Tian XJ, Donnenberg VS, Watson AM, Zhang J, Stabile LP, et al. Targeting the temporal dynamics of hypoxia-induced tumor-secreted factors halts tumor migration. Cancer Research. 2019;**79**(11):2962-2977. DOI: 10.1158/0008-5472.CAN-18-3151

[39] Yin M, Tissari M, Tamminen J, Ylivinkka I, Ronty M, von Nandelstadh P, et al. Gremlin-1 is a key regulator of the invasive cell phenotype in mesothelioma. Oncotarget. 2017;**8**(58):98280-98297. DOI: 10.18632/oncotarget.21550

[40] Ying S, Jiang Z, He X, Yu M, Chen R, Chen J, et al. Serum HMGB1 as a potential biomarker for patients with asbestos-related diseases. Disease Markers. 2017;**2017**:5756102. DOI: 10.1155/2017/5756102

[41] Villanova T, Gesmundo I, Audrito V, Vitale N, Silvagno F, Musuraca C, et al. Antagonists of growth hormone-releasing

hormone (GHRH) inhibit the growth of human malignant pleural mesothelioma. Proceedings of the National Academy of Sciences of the United States of America. 2019;**116**(6):2226-2231. DOI: 10.1073/pnas.1818865116

[42] Muscella A, Cossa LG, Vetrugno C, Antonaci G, Marsigliante S. Adenosine diphosphate regulates MMP2 and MMP9 activity in malignant mesothelioma cells. Annals of the New York Academy of Sciences. 2018;**1431**(1):72-84. DOI: 10.1111/nyas.13922

[43] Cheng S, Xu Y, Shi Z, Lin Y, Hoang CD, Zhang X. Overexpression of micro ribonucleic acid-591 inhibits cell proliferation and invasion of malignant pleural mesothelioma cells. Thoracic Cancer. 2016;7(3):340-347. DOI: 10.1111/1759-7714.12336

[44] Husain AN, Colby TV, Ordonez NG, Allen TC, Attanoos RL, Beasley MB, et al. Guidelines for pathologic diagnosis of malignant mesothelioma 2017 update of the consensus statement from the international mesothelioma interest group. Archives of Pathology & Laboratory Medicine. 2018;**142**(1):89-108. DOI: 10.5858/arpa.2017-0124-RA

[45] Davidson B, Stavnes HT, Hellesylt E, Hager T, Zeppa P, Pinamonti M, et al. MMP-7 is a highly specific negative marker for benign and malignant mesothelial cells in serous effusions. Human Pathology. 2016;**47**(1):104-108. DOI: 10.1016/j.humpath.2015.08.020

[46] Ali G, Borrelli N, Riccardo G, Proietti A, Pelliccioni S, Niccoli C, et al. Differential expression of extracellular matrix constituents and cell adhesion molecules between malignant pleural mesothelioma and mesothelial hyperplasia. Journal of Thoracic Oncology. 2013;**8**(11):1389-1395. DOI: 10.1097/JTO.0b013e3182a59f45

[47] Crispi S, Calogero RA, Santini M, Mellone P, Vincenzi B, Citro G, et al. Global gene expression profiling of human pleural mesotheliomas: Identification of matrix metalloproteinase 14 (MMP-14) as potential tumour target. PLoS ONE. 2009;**4**(9):e7016. DOI: 10.1371/journal.pone.0007016

[48] Ohar JA, Cheung M, Talarchek J, Howard SE, Howard TD, Hesdorffer M, et al. Germline BAP1 mutational landscape of asbestos-exposed malignant mesothelioma patients with family history of cancer. Cancer Research. 2016;**76**(2):206-215. DOI: 10.1158/0008-5472.CAN-15-0295

[49] Leblay N, Lepretre F, Le Stang N, Gautier-Stein A, Villeneuve L, Isaac S, et al. BAP1 is altered by copy number loss, mutation, and/or loss of protein expression in more than 70% of malignant peritoneal mesotheliomas. Journal of Thoracic Oncology. 2017;**12**(4):724-733. DOI: 10.1016/j.jtho.2016.12.019

[50] Baumann F, Flores E, Napolitano A, Kanodia S, Taioli E, Pass H, et al. Mesothelioma patients with germline BAP1 mutations have 7-fold improved long-term survival. Carcinogenesis. 2015;**36**(1):76-81. DOI: 10.1093/carcin/bgu227

[51] Strbac D, Goricar K, Dolzan V, Kovac V. Matrix metalloproteinases polymorphisms as prognostic biomarkers in malignant pleural mesothelioma. Disease Markers. 2017;**2017**:8069529. DOI: 10.1155/2017/8069529

[52] Strbac D, Goricar K, Dolzan V, Kovac V. Matrix metalloproteinases polymorphisms as baseline risk predictors in malignant pleural mesothelioma. Radiology and Oncology. 2018;**52**(2):160-166. DOI: 10.2478/raon-2018-0005